Introduction to Sports Medicine

quantum scientific publishing

Introduction to Sports Medicine

Susan M. Carlson

Carly Ann Pietrzyk, PhD

quantum scientific publishing

Introduction to Sports Medicine

ISBN-13: 978-1493697502
ISBN-10: 1493697501

Published by quantum scientific publishing

Pittsburgh, PA | Copyright © 2013

All rights reserved. Permission in writing must be obtained from the publisher before any part of this work may be reproduced or transmitted in any form, including photocopying and recording.

Cover design by Scott Sheariss

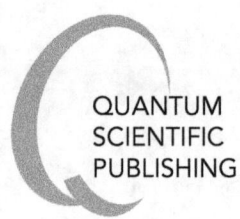

Unit One

Section 1.1 – Introduction to Sports Medicine 10

Section 1.2 – Careers in Sports Medicine 15

Section 1.3 – Joint Basics 21

Section 1.4 – Rehabilitation Theories 31

Section 1.5 – Range of Motion 35

Section 1.6 – Muscle Stiffness 39

Section 1.7 – Heart Rate 43

Section 1.8 – Body Mass Index 47

Section 1.9 – The Five-Level Model of Body Composition 51

Section 1.10 – Power, Speed and Agility 59

Section 1.11 – The Functional Movement Screen 63

Section 1.12 – Stretching 69

Section 1.13 – Corrective Exercise Program 75

Section 1.14 – Muscle Tissue Quality 79

Section 1.15 – Nutritional Supplements 83

Unit Two

Section 2.1 – The Cardiovascular System 92

Section 2.2 – Measuring Cardiovascular Function 97

Section 2.3 – The Respiratory System 101

Section 2.4 – Lung Volume 103

Section 2.5 – The Skeletal System 107

Section 2.6 – Bone Tissue and Bone Health 111

Section 2.7 – The Stress-Strain Curve 115

Section 2.8 – Joints and Levers 119

Section 2.9 – The Muscular System 123

Section 2.10 – The Central Nervous System 127

Section 2.11 – The FIT Principle 131

Section 2.12 – Power, Strength, and Endurance 135

Section 2.13 – Interval Training: Aerobic and Anaerobic Conditioning 139

Section 2.14 – Sets and Repetitions 143

Section 2.15 – Thibaudeau's Six Training Programs 145

Unit Three

- Section 3.1 – Brain Injuries   150
- Section 3.2 – Spinal Cord Injuries   155
- Section 3.3 – Assessment and Treatment of Spinal Cord Injuries   159
- Section 3.4 – The Shoulder and Shoulder Injuries   163
- Section 3.5 – The Elbow and Elbow Injuries   167
- Section 3.6 – The Body's Core   169
- Section 3.7 – The Wrist   173
- Section 3.8 – The Hand   177
- Section 3.9 – The Spinal Column   181
- Section 3.10 – The Hip   187
- Section 3.11 – Structure of the Knee   189
- Section 3.12 – Knee Injuries   191
- Section 3.13 – The Ankle and Ankle Injuries   193
- Section 3.14 – The Foot and Foot Injuries   197
- Section 3.15 – Osteoarthritis   201

Appendix

- Unit One Answer Key   206
- Unit Two Answer Key   210
- Unit Three Answer Key   216

Unit One

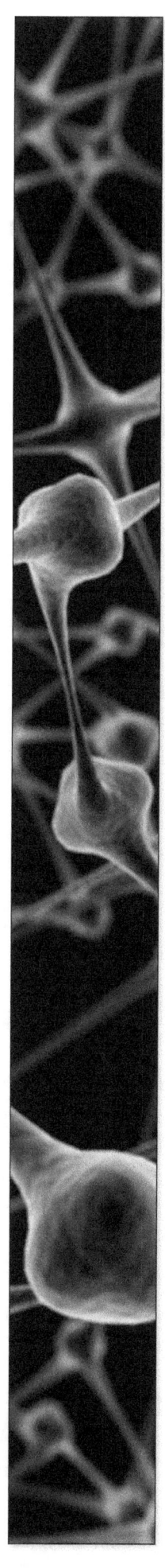

Section 1.1 – Introduction to Sports Medicine   10

Section 1.2 – Careers in Sports Medicine   15

Section 1.3 – Joint Basics   21

Section 1.4 – Rehabilitation Theories   31

Section 1.5 – Range of Motion   35

Section 1.6 – Muscle Stiffness   39

Section 1.7 – Heart Rate   43

Section 1.8 – Body Mass Index   47

Section 1.9 – The Five-Level Model of Body Composition   51

Section 1.10 – Power, Speed and Agility   59

Section 1.11 – The Functional Movement Screen   63

Section 1.12 – Stretching   69

Section 1.13 – Corrective Exercise Program   75

Section 1.14 – Muscle Tissue Quality   79

Section 1.15 – Nutritional Supplements   83

Section 1.1 – Introduction to Sports Medicine

Section Objective

- Define sports medicine

What Is Sports Medicine?

Sports medicine is using medicine to prevent, diagnose and treat sports injuries. Sports medicine includes research (study), and practice (application) of medical principles to diagnose, treat and prevent injury, as well as in sports training and athletic performance.

Sports medicine professionals specialize in preventing, diagnosing and treating athlete injuries. They may also focus on athletic performance and sports training. There are many different specialties in sports medicine. These specialties require different levels of education, experience and certification. A list of some sports medicine specialties is below.

Field	Education	Certification	License
Athletic Trainer	Bachelor's degree from an accredited program required to take the NATA certification exam.	National Athletic Trainers' Association	Required in most states.
Biomechanicist	Masters degree	n/a	n/a
Chiropractor	Doctor of Chiropractic	National Board of Chiropractic Examiners	Yes
Exercise Physiologist	Bachelor's degree in a related field	American College of Sports Medicine	n/a
Massage Therapist	Accredited massage therapy program	National Certification Board for Therapeutic Massage and Bodywork	Yes
Occupational Therapist	Bachelor's degree + 2-3 years experience.	National certification exam	Yes
Physical Therapist	Master's Degree	National Certification exam	Yes
Personal Trainer	Bachelor's degree	American College of Sports Medicine	No
Sports Physician	Medical Doctor	Yes – the certification agency depends upon the speciality.	Yes

Teacher	Bachelor's degree or higher	State exam	Yes
Strength and Conditioning Coach	Masters Degree	National Strength and Conditioning Association	No
Sports Psychologist	Masters Degree	Yes	Yes
Sports Nutritionist	Bachelor's degree in dietetics + 9 month American Dietetics Association internship	American Dietetics Association	No

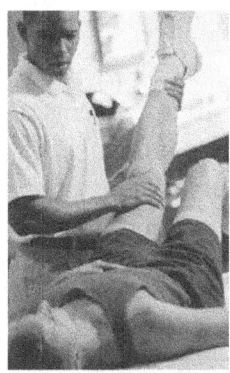

Leg exam
Image courtesy of the National Institutes of Health

Sports medicine professionals work in a wide variety of organizations, including schools, hospitals and professional sports teams. The chart below shows the industries in which athletic trainers work.

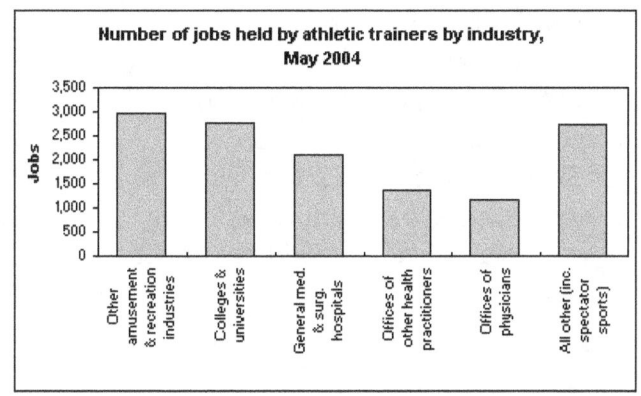

Courtesy of the US Bureau of Labor Statistics

High schools with sports teams usually have a trainer on staff to help the student athletes prevent and treat sports-related injuries. University sports teams often have more than one athletic trainer. This depends on the number and size of the teams at the university. A football team, for example, is likely to have several trainers to treat the players and help them recover from injured knees and ankles, head trauma, and other football-related injuries. Professional sports teams have sports medicine physicians and trainers on staff. The athletes playing on this level sustain significant injuries and need to be able to recover fully as quickly as possible to continue contributing to the team. Sports medicine professionals in hospitals repair injuries and help athletes recover fully by providing physical therapy and medication to help the healing process.

The History Of Sports Medicine

Sports medicine is an ancient field. The Arthava-Veda, an ancient medical book from India, described the first uses of therapeutic exercises. This book dates back to about 800-1000 B.C. That is about 3,000 years ago! More recent advances in the field include the Tommy John surgery, which is an elbow repair technique developed by Dr. Frank Jobe in the 1970s to treat baseball players. The Tommy John surgery is an elbow ligament replacement. Currently, 83% of patients recover fully and are able to resume pitching. Other advances in sports medicine include improvements in preventing, diagnosing and managing concussions. The largest improvements are in protective gear, such as mouth guards and helmets, which prevent a huge number of concussions each year. Arthroscopic surgery has improved the treatment of sports injury and speeded recovery. This is because the surgery is much less invasive than standard surgery. It is used to do certain joint repairs and allows athletes to enter rehabilitation programs within a few days of surgery. A recent improvement is the introduction of hypothermia therapy for suspected spinal cord injuries. This treatment seems to limit swelling that might otherwise cause permanent damage. As medical technology advances, athletes benefit from the application of that technology to injury prevention, treatment and rehabilitation.

The field of sports medicine has grown a lot since 1928, when the Federation of Sports Medicine was established to provide medical care to the athletes competing in the St. Moritz winter Olympics. The American Medical Association established a committee on Injuries in Sports in 1951. Following that, the American College of Sports Medicine was established in 1954. ACSM is now the largest of all of the sports medicine organizations. The American Orthopedic Society for Sports Medicine was founded in 1971. An educational organization, the National Athletic Trainers Association, was established in 1950 to provide education to athletic trainers.

Sports Medicine In Modern Life

Sports medicine has affected you whether or not you are an athlete. The athletic shoes you wear are designed to minimize injury. Tennis and basketball shoes help prevent injuries related to sprinting, stopping quickly, and turning. Running shoes reduce the impact of running on your feet, ankles, knees and hips. The braces, helmets and other protective gear worn by athletes are designed to protect them from injury while still allowing them to compete in their sports.

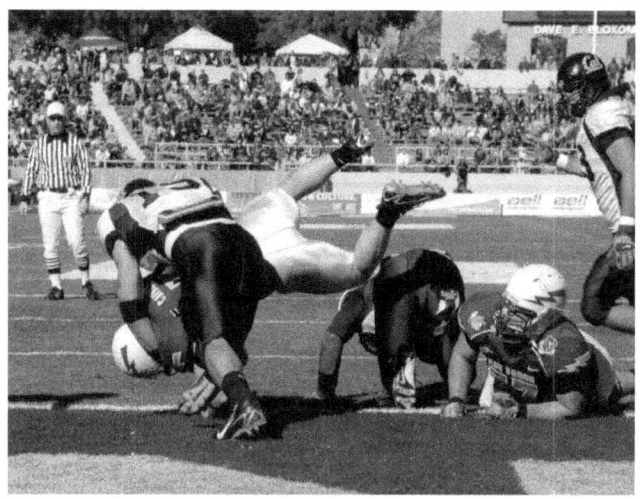

Air Force Academy quarterback Shaun Carney (5) dives into the end zone for a touchdown during the Armed Forces Bowl football game in Fort Worth, Texas, Dec. 31. Carney's game ended with an unfortunate knee injury late in the third quarter as California defeated the Air Force 42 to 36.
Lt. Col. William Thurmond, USA
Photo Courtesy of U.S. Army

The knowledge and practices developed for sports medicine are used by physical therapists to treat injuries, whether or not the patient is an athlete. A knee injury is a knee injury, regardless of how it happened. Therefore, it is logical that treatments developed for an athlete will work for a non-athlete.

Summary

The field of sports medicine includes a wide variety of disciplines. These range from athletic trainers to surgeons and researchers to teachers. Sports medicine goes back to about 1000 B.C., when therapeutic exercises were included in the Arthava-Veda, an ancient Indian book. Researchers and clinicians are constantly developing new approaches to preventing and treating athletic injuries. This knowledge is used to help everyone who has those injuries, whether or not they are athletes.

Concept Reinforcement

1. List three specialties in sports medicine.

2. Explain why the Federation of Sports Medicine was established.

3. Describe how gains in sports medicine affect non-athletes and athletes alike.

Section 1.2 – Careers in Sports Medicine

Section Objective

- Describe several different careers in the sports medicine field

Careers

Sports medicine is a broad field that includes many different careers. When you think of sports medicine, you probably think of an athletic trainer first. There are many other professions in sports medicine. These include physicians, coaches, psychologists, nutritionists, and many others.

Athletic Trainer

An athletic trainer is in direct contact with the athletes and helps them stay healthy as they are doing their sports. Athletic trainers are very important to athletes because they understand the body and how it works, know how to prevent injury, and finally how to treat an injury and help the athlete recover. Athletic trainers are at the games and usually one of the first to respond if someone is hurt on the field.

A certified athletic trainer usually has at least a bachelor's degree. The degree could be in athletic training, physical education, education science, or health. They must have a thorough understanding of the human body, as well as nutrition and psychology. In order to become a certified athletic trainer (ATC), one must meet the requirements for certification established by the National Athletic Trainers' Association Board of Certification, Inc. (NATABOC). The certification exam has three parts. The written portion tests general knowledge. The practical section evaluates hands-on skills. The written simulation tests the trainer's ability to assess an injury and make correct treatment decisions. The key areas covered in the exam are prevention of athletic injuries; recognition, evaluation and immediate care of sports injuries; rehabilitation and reconditioning of sports injuries; health care administration; and professional development and responsibility.

Sports Medicine Physician

A sports medicine physician specializes in sport and exercise-related injuries. These doctors promote lifelong wellness and fitness. They also work with athletes to prevent and treat illness and injury. The sports medicine physician is usually the leader of the sports medicine team, which may include other physicians, athletic trainers, nutritionists, physical therapists, coaches, and others. These professionals are well trained in anatomy and physiology, as well as in how to treat acute injuries (a broken bone, for example) and overuse injuries. They also receive training on head injuries, nutrition, managing chronic illnesses, and other relevant disciplines.

A sports medicine physician has extensive education. A medical doctor degree is required, along with a three-year residency, typically in family medicine or orthopedics. Some even obtain specialized sports medicine training and accreditation. Physicians must also pass national boards in order to practice law.

Orthopedic Surgeon

Orthopedic surgeons specialize in repairing the musculoskeletal system. Athletes often sustain injuries to their joints and muscles that require surgical repair. The injury could be the result of overuse or an acute injury caused by a fall or collision. Orthopedic surgeons repair joints and pin broken bones together.

The educational requirements for an orthopedic surgeon are the same as for the sports medicine physician. The only difference is the type of residency required.

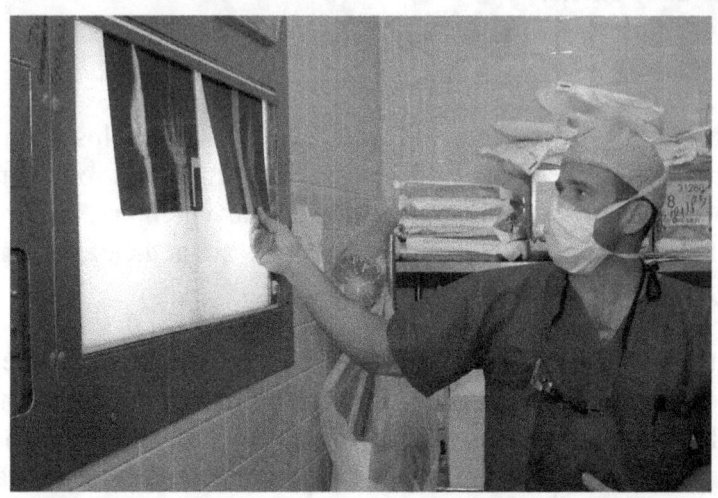

Army Lt. Col. (Dr.) Martin Baechler, an orthopedic surgeon from Walter Reed Army Medical Center, examines a patient's X-ray at Hospital Escuela in Tegucigalpa, Honduras, during MEDRETE (U.S. Army).

Coach

An athletic coach organizes and teaches athletes in individual and team sports. They plan strategy, inspire players, enforce the rules, and train the athletes to play the game. Coaches coach teams or individuals, depending upon the athlete's sport. Coaches also play an important role as a counselor and advisor to the athletes. Coaches lead the team and set an example for the athletes. Coaches may be volunteers or paid. Little League coaches are volunteers. High school, college and pro-sport coaches are paid professionals.

The educational requirements for coaches vary based on the level at which they are coaching. Entry-level positions may only require knowing how to play the sport. High school coaches who are not teachers may have to meet specific state certification requirements in order to coach.

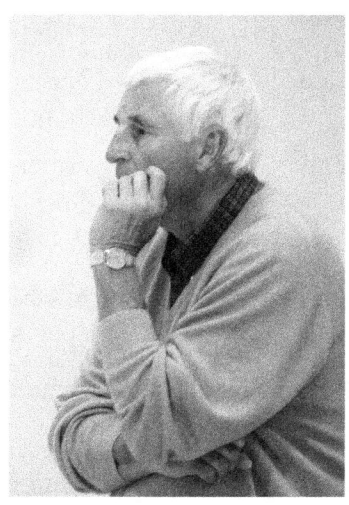

Coach Bobby Knight observing his team at practice.

Physical Therapist

Physical therapists help athletes regain function after an injury. They may also work with athletes to help prevent injury. Specifically, physical therapists work with patients to restore function, improve mobility, relieve pain and try to prevent or limit physical problems from an injury or illness from becoming permanent. As with sports medicine physicians, physical therapists promote overall health and fitness.

The educational requirements for a physical therapist are a master's degree from an accredited physical therapy program. A physical therapist must pass state and national licensing exams in order to obtain a license to practice. Physical therapy students receive instruction in the classroom, laboratory and in the clinic.

Field	Education	Certification	License
Athletic Trainer	Bachelor's degree from an accredited program required to take the NATA certification exam.	National Athletic Trainers' Association	Required in most states.
Biomechanicist	Masters degree	n/a	n/a
Chiropractor	Doctor of Chiropractic	National Board of Chiropractic Examiners	Yes
Exercise Physiologist	Bachelor's degree in a related field	American College of Sports Medicine	n/a
Massage Therapist	Accredited massage therapy program	National Certification Board for Therapeutic Massage and Bodywork	Yes
Occupational Therapist	Bachelor's degree + 2-3 years experience.	National certification exam	Yes

Field	Education	Certification	License
Physical Therapist	Master's Degree	National Certification exam	Yes
Personal Trainer	Bachelor's degree	American College of Sports Medicine	No
Sports Physician	Medical Doctor	Yes – the certification agency depends upon the speciality.	Yes
Teacher	Bachelor's degree or higher	State exam	Yes
Strength and Conditioning Coach	Masters Degree	National Strength and Conditioning Association	No
Sports Psychologist	Masters Degree	Yes	Yes
Sports Nutritionist	Bachelor's degree in dietetics + 9 month American Dietetics Association internship	American Dietetics Association	No
Orthopedic Surgeon	Medical Doctor	American Board of Orthopedic Surgery	Yes
Coach	Varies – depending on the level	No	No
Kinesiologist	Bachelor's Degree	Optional – American Council on Exercise; American College of Sports Medicine; National Strength and Conditioning Association	No

Sport Psychologist

A sport psychologist studies the psychological and mental factors that influence sports performance, as well as those factors influenced by participation in sports. They apply their knowledge to understand how participation in sports improves personal development, well being, and athlete motivation.

A sport psychologist goes through extensive training, often obtaining a doctorate degree. It is possible to practice sports psychology with a bachelor's degree, although there are few jobs at this level. There are many more jobs at the master's degree level.

Kinesiologist

Kinesiology is the study of movement. In terms of sports medicine, kinesiology refers to the study of athletic movement. A kinesiologist works with athletes to improve movement patterns. This is important for athletic performance, as well as preventing injury. Proper movement is important in injury prevention. Kinesiologists also play a role in developing new training techniques, using muscle testing as a diagnostic tool, and designing new equipment.

A kinesiologist has a minimum of a bachelor's degree. There are optional certifications available for those who want to teach. The American Council on Exercise, the American College of Sports Medicine, and the National Strength and Conditioning Association all offer certifications. Advanced degrees are required for certain research fields.

Massage Therapist

A massage therapist works with athletes to ensure flexibility and relaxation. Massage therapists are able to relax muscles, which allows blood to deliver oxygen more efficiently and may also help decrease pain.

A massage therapist is trained in one or more types of massage (Swedish, deep tissue, trigger point, shiatsu, etc.). Training programs include instruction in massage, as well as training (usually 500 hours) and topics related to massage. Many states require massage therapists to be licensed. There are also certification programs.

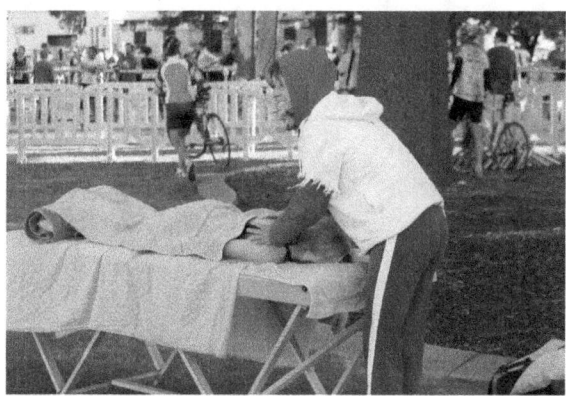

Massage therapist working at a Triathlon in Fremantle, Western Australia, Australia.
Image by Bob Whitehead from Perth, Australia

Summary

There are many more careers in sports medicine than we have covered here. We discussed several different careers with different educational and certification requirements. The people who follow these careers all play an important role in maintaining the health of athletes. The sports medicine physician is usually the leader of the sports medicine team. Each team member brings a unique skill set and expertise that is essential.

Concept Reinforcement

1. Describe the role of a coach on the sports medicine team.

2. Describe the role of the massage therapist on the sports medicine team.

3. Explain the educational requirements for a certified athletic trainer.

4. Explain kinesiology and its role in sports medicine.

Section 1.3 – Joint Basics

Section Objective

- Explain the joint-by-joint theory and discuss the long term impact of repetitive motion

The Body

The human body is made to move. If we are healthy, we move properly. If we are not healthy, we are able to change our movement patterns to adapt to the injury or illness we are coping with. The joint-by-joint theory is a way of explaining how joints needs to function for healthy, pain-free movement.

Joints

The skeleton is the frame of our bodies. All of the muscles, tendons, and other tissues rely on the strength of the skeleton. The joints are the connecting points between the bones that allow movement. Some joints move only in one plane (think about the knee), while others have a much wider range of motion (the shoulder). The health of each joint depends upon the health of the surrounding joints. For example, the knee joint depends on both the ankle and hip working properly in order for the knee to remain healthy.

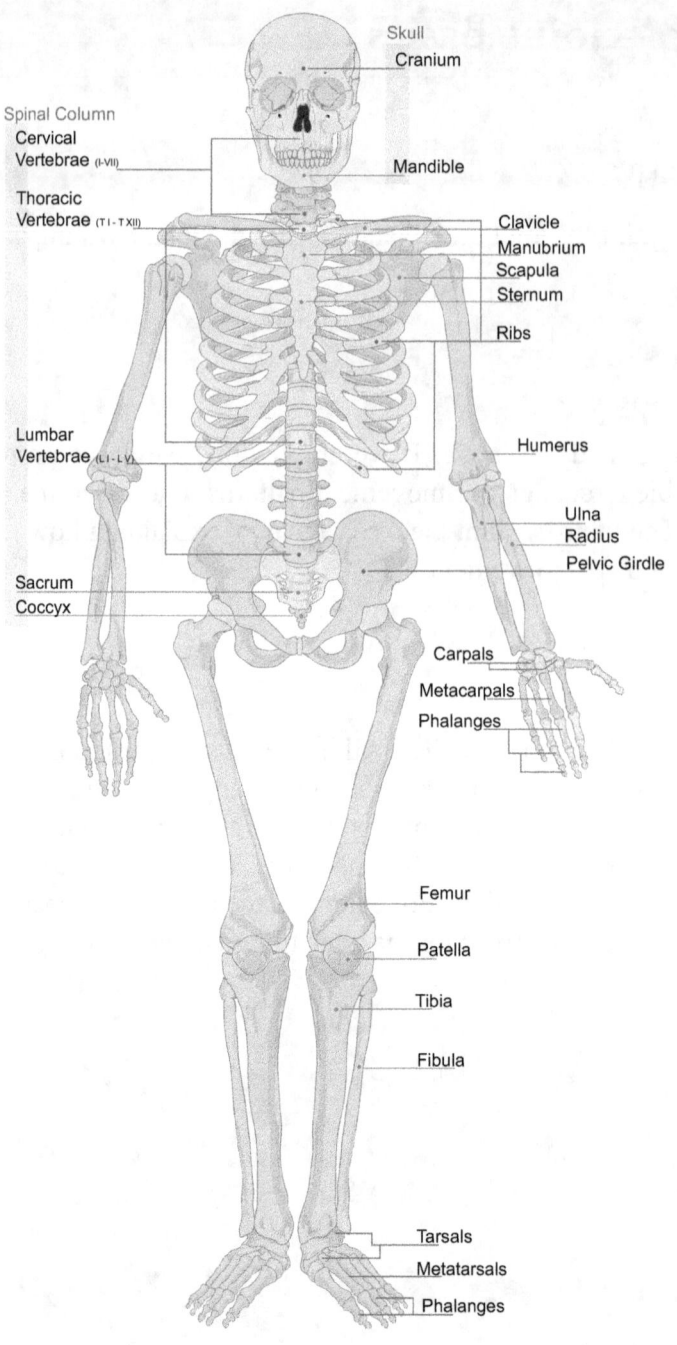

The Joint-by-Joint Theory

The Joint-by-Joint Theory states that the joints of the human body are organized so they alternate between stability and mobility. For example, a mobile joint (the ankle, for example), supports a stable joint (the knee). If the ankle does not move properly, it will affect the knee, which may then develop an injury.

Joint-by-Joint Theory

Neck to Arms		Neck to Toes	
Cervical Spine (neck)	Stable	Cervical Spine (neck)	Stable
Thoracic Spine (middle back)	Mobile	Thoracic Spine (middle back)	Mobile
Scapula (shoulder blades)	Stable	Lumbar Spine (lower back)	Stable
Gleno-humeral Joint (shoulder)	Mobile	Hip	Mobile
Elbow	Stable	Knee	Stable
Wrist	Mobile	Talo-Crural Joint (Ankle)	Mobile
Thumb	Stable	Sub-Talar Joint (heel) and mid-foot	Stable
		Big Toe	Mobile

The basic theory is if you lose function in a joint, it will affect the joint(s) above the injured one. Therefore, pain in one joint may be the result of a problem in another joint.

Let's look at some examples, starting with the ankle.

The Ankle

You often hear of basketball players having ankle injuries because of all the jumping they do. The basketball shoes they wear have a lot of ankle support in them, which should help prevent injury. However, since the ankle is a mobile joint, this extra support may actually be transferring the stress of the landing to the knee, causing knee problems for the athlete.

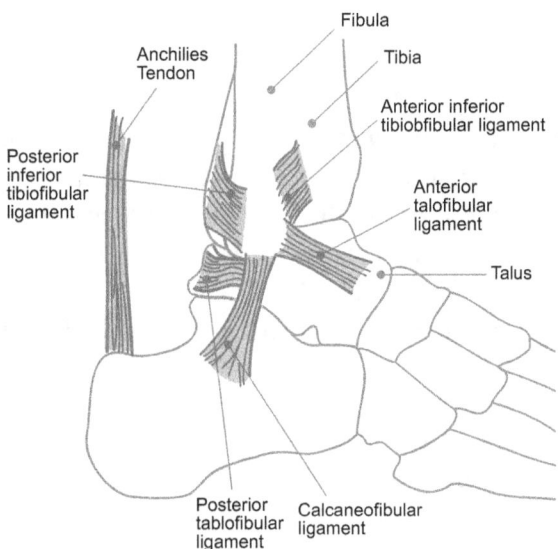

As you can see from this image, the ankle is a very complex joint. When jumping, the ankle has the mobility to absorb the shock of the landing. When the ankle is supported too much by shoes or tape, it is not able to move like it needs to absorb the shock. When that happens, the shock goes up the leg to the knee, potentially causing knee problems.

The Knee

The knee is a stable joint. It moves forward and backward like a hinge. The knee joint does not move side to side unless it is seriously injured. In the joint-by-joint theory, the knee is a stable joint. If the ankle or hip is not moving correctly, the knee may be forced to be more mobile to adapt to the problems in the hip or ankle. This leads to knee problems, often involving the ligaments and tendons, because of the incorrect movement. Can you see why basketball players might develop knee problems if their ankles are not allowed to move properly?

Definitions

Patella = knee

Medial = Inside

Lateral = Outside

Anterior = Front

Collateral = related to

Meniscus = a cushion in the joint

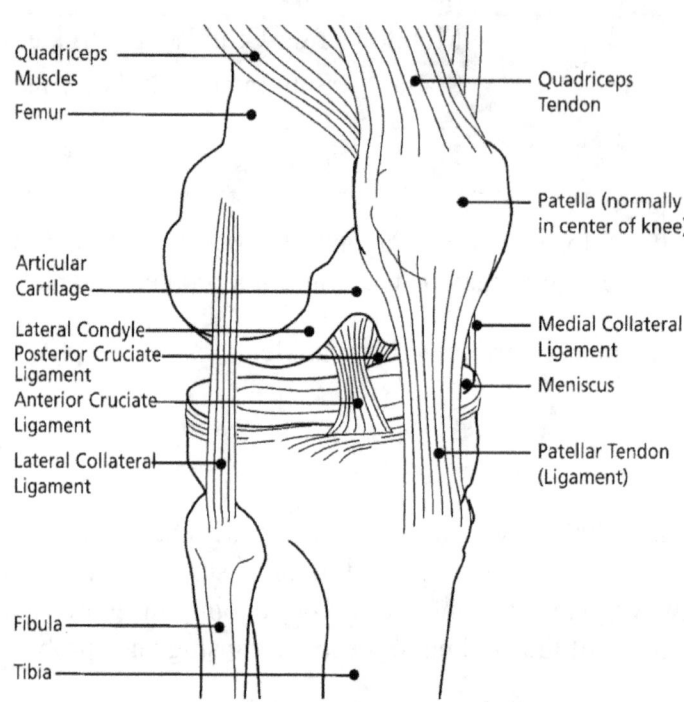

The location of knee pain can help identify the problem. Pain on the front of the knee can be due to bursitis, arthritis, or softening of the patella cartilage. Pain on the sides of the knee is commonly related to injuries to the ligaments, arthritis, or tears to the meniscuses. Pain in the back of the knee can be caused by arthritis or cysts, known as Baker's cysts. Baker's cysts are an accumulation of joint fluid (synovial fluid) that forms behind the knee. Overall knee pain can be due to bursitis, arthritis, tears in the ligaments, osteoarthritis of the joint, or infection.

Instability, or giving way, is also another common knee problem. Instability is usually associated with damage or problems with the meniscuses, collateral ligaments, or patella tracking.

The Hip

The hip is the one joint that must be both mobile and stable. The hip, like the shoulder, may be both immobile and unstable at the same time. It may also be both mobile and stable at the same time. If the hip is healthy, it has good flexibility and range of motion. It also has the strength to support its movements. Hip immobility is caused by lack of flexibility and lack of motion. Hip instability is due to weakness or not following a comprehensive lower body training program. Both hip instability and immobility cause movement problems at the lumbar (lower) spine.

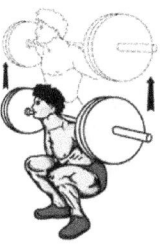

Let's look at an example – the squat. The hips are very involved in the squat motion. If the hips are not flexible or stable enough to perform the squat motion properly, the strain moves up to the lumbar spine. Remember that the lumbar spine is a stable joint. If the hips are unable to move enough to perform a squat, the lumbar spine is forced to be more mobile, which can lead to back pain and injury. In this particular situation, the lack of mobility of the hip leads the back to compensate for the lack of mobility in the hip. This can then lead to even less mobility in the hip, which causes a vicious cycle of poor movement and compensatory movement.

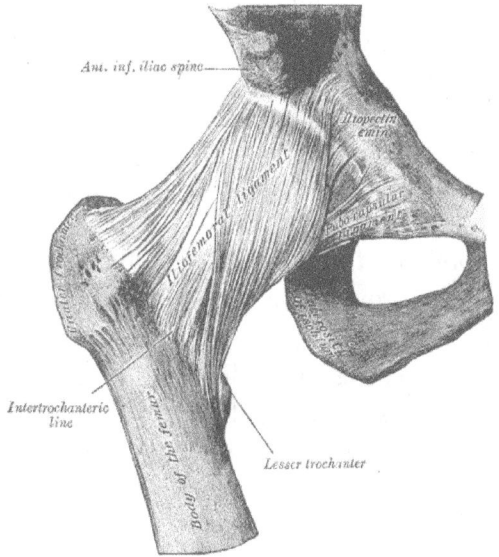

Weakness in the hip can place additional stress on the knee, as well. If the hip joint is unable to rotate to allow for up and down movement, the knee and lower back will adapt to allow that movement to occur. This adaptation forces the joints to be more mobile than they should be, which can lead to injury. It is important to remember that muscular strength and flexibility are key to proper joint movement.

The Lumbar Spine

Different parts of the spine are named based on location and movement. The lumbar spine is the lower spine. When you hear people complain about low back pain, they are talking about pain in the lumbar spine. In the joint-by-joint theory, the lumbar spine is the stable part of the spine. In fact, when you hear discussions of developing the core, part of the discussion is strengthening the muscles around the lumbar spine to help it remain stable.

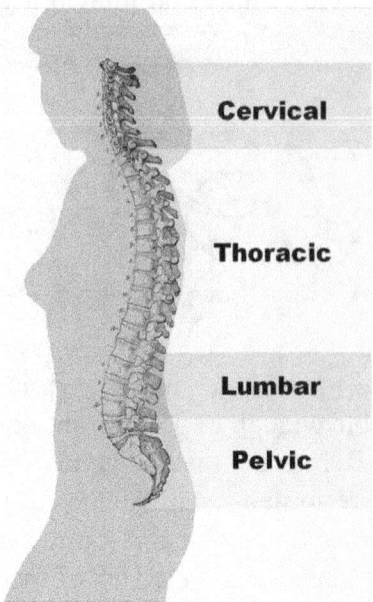

It is very important to use proper form when doing squats or other exercises that involve the back. The lumbar spine is prone to injury if you do not use good form. Once you have a lower back injury, it is very difficult to fully recover from that injury and you may end up with life-long problems.

Thoracic Spine

The thoracic spine is the mobile part of the spine that allows us to rotate our torsos. Not as much is known about how to improve thoracic spine mobility as is known for other joints. Practicing yoga may help improve thoracic spine mobility. Yoga focuses on flexibility, strength and extension of the muscles, as well as proper alignment of the body. Another benefit of yoga is that you do the work yourself instead of having the work done to you by a therapist or trainer. This allows you to work at your own pace to develop your flexibility and strength.

The Scapulo-Thoracic Joint

The next joint we will talk about in the joint-by-joint theory is the scapulo-thoracic joint, which is a stable joint. This joint is not commonly know by this name, but is where your shoulder blade connects with the torso. The scapulo-thoracic joint is the interface between the shoulder and the rest of the body. The shoulder blade is in your back, but the top curves over the top of the shoulder and connects to the torso with tendons.

This joint is very important for lifting with the arms and is usually under-exercised. In order for the scapulo-thoracic joint to be strong, the muscles surrounding it must be strong.

The lower trapezius muscle, which connects to the spine and up to the shoulder joint, is usually under exercised. This muscle can be strengthened by doing rowing exercises, either in a boat or in a seated position.

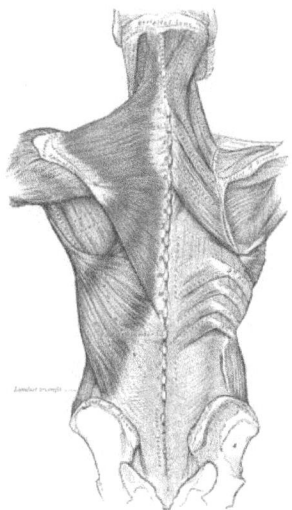

This image shows the trapezius muscle. The upper part of the muscle is usually well developed in power lifters and other athletes, but the lower part of the muscle is often underdeveloped, which can lead to shoulder problems.

The Gleno-Humeral Joint (Shoulder)

The gleno-humeral joint is the final joint we will discuss in the joint-by-joint theory. The shoulder is similar to the hip because it is a very mobile joint, but must also be stable to perform lifting motions. Shoulder mobility is supported by the stable scapulo-thoracic joint. If the shoulder joint is not properly supported when performing movements such as throwing, the shoulder is susceptible to injury. The muscles surrounding the shoulder can be strengthened by using specific exercises that increase both strength and mobility in the joint.

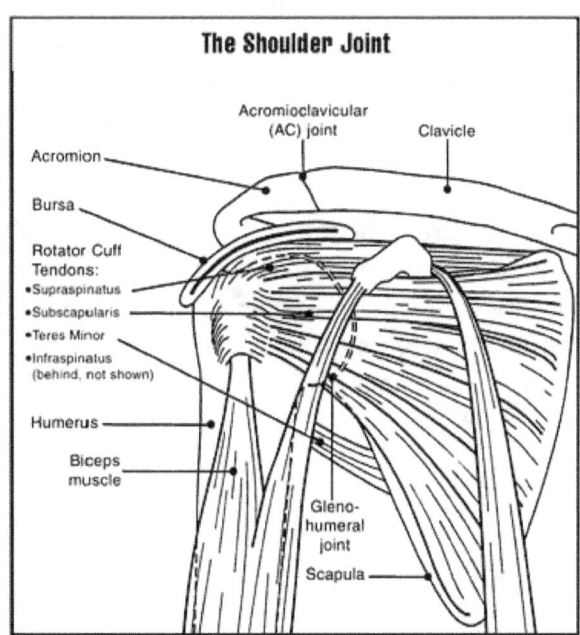

When tendons become trapped under the acromion, the rigid bony arch of the shoulder blade, it can cause shoulder pain called impingement syndrome. The tendons become compressed, damaged, and inflamed leading to rotator cuff tendinitis. This can occur from general wear and tear as you get older, or from an activity that requires constant use of the shoulder like baseball pitching, or from an injury.

The Impact Of Long-Term Repetitive Motion

As you can see, proper movement is essential to joint health. Correcting movement early prevents long-term injury. Repetitive motion injury is very common in the US, making up over 50% of sports-related injuries. The most common types of repetitive motion injuries are tendinitis and bursitis. Tendinitis is an inflammation of the tendon. Tendons connect muscles to bone and allow all the joints in the body to move. Bursitis is inflammation of the bursa sac in a joint. The bursa sac is a small pouch found in joints at points of friction. Bursae cushion or lubricate the areas of friction.

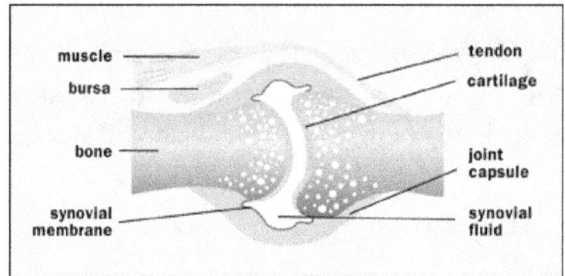

Normal Joint: In a normal joint (where two bones come together), the muscle, bursa and tendon support the bone and aid movement. The synovial membrane (an inner lining) releases a slippery fluid into the joint space. Cartilage covers the bone ends, absorbing shocks and keeping the bones from rubbing together when the joint moves. Image Courtesy of the General Services Administration, US Government

Repetitive motion injuries are the result of microscopic tears in the tissues. If the body is unable to repair the tears as fast as they are made, the tissues become inflamed (swollen), which can lead to pain. There are many causes of repetitive motion injuries, including repetitive activity, trauma, crystal deposits in the tissue that cause tears, friction in the joint, and systemic diseases, such as arthritis.

If these injuries are not treated properly, they can lead to a lack of mobility. This can become a permanent condition if the body is unable to heal itself. It is possible to prevent repetitive motion injuries by following a proper warm-up and cool-down routine, using proper form in your movement, working to maintain your range of motion, and properly treating symptoms when they first occur.

Summary

The body is a complex machine supported by the skeletal system. The joints in the skeleton allow us to move to perform both everyday activities and competitive sports. The joint-by-joint theory describes the relationships between the stable and mobile joints, as well as the movement problems that can develop when a joint is injured or not moving properly. Long-term repetition of improper movement can lead to reduced mobility in joints and chronic pain. Repetitive motion injuries are treatable and preventable.

Concept Reinforcement

1. Explain the role of a joint in the human body.

2. Describe the joint-by-joint theory.

3. Discuss how pain in one joint may indicate a problem in another joint.

4. List two causes of repetitive motion injuries.

Section 1.4 – Rehabilitation Theories

Section Objective

- List the four progressions in rehabilitation theories

Rehabilitation

The human body, while made to move, is also prone to injury. This occurs when we have traumatic injury to the body, for example a collision or fall. Injury also occurs as a result of improper training or faulty movement.

Dr. Shirley Sahrmann has led a fundamental change in how we approach rehabilitation after illness or injury. Everything we do to help people recover is based on what we know about the body and how it moves.

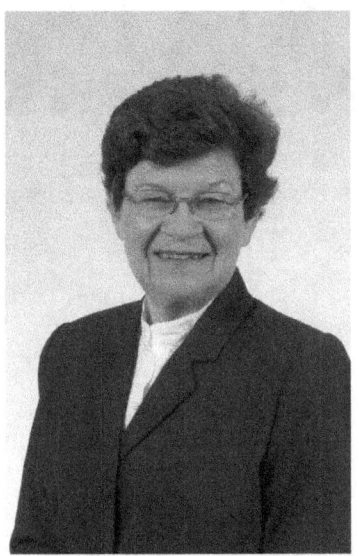

Dr. Shirley A. Sahrmann, PT, PhD, FAPTA

First Rehabilitation Theory

Dr. Sahrmann developed her first theory by studying people who have polio. Polio does not affect many people in the US any more because the disease is prevented with polio vaccines. However, there are still people who had polio before vaccines were available and are dealing with the long-term results of the disease.

People with polio develop muscle weakness. The muscle weakness then leads to faulty movement patterns. These faulty movement patterns cause pain and injury to other parts of the body.

Dr. Sahrmann studied the movement of polio patients. These patients showed muscle weakness and the related faulty movement. She deduced that the muscle is the driving force of human movement. Injured muscle must heal completely before trying to strengthen it with an exercise program. If the muscles are not working properly, it does not matter how healthy the joints are because we will not move properly, if at all. As a result of this finding, patients are given strength tests as part of rehabilitation. The results of the strength tests are key to developing the correct rehabilitation program.

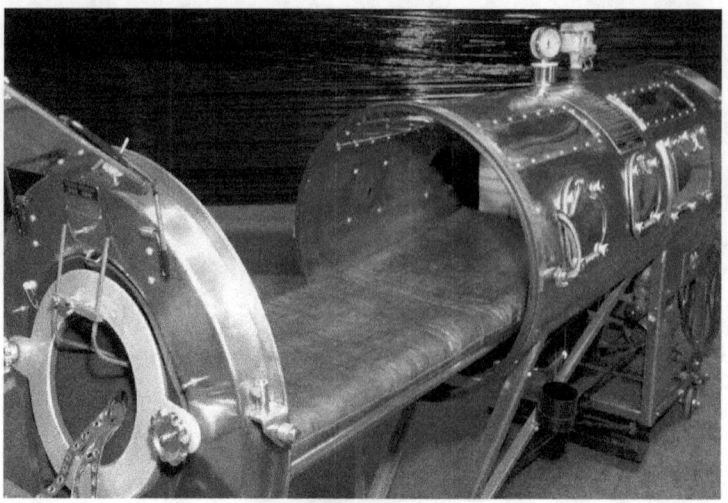

This photograph shows an opened artificial respirator commonly known as the iron lung. Polio patients of the 1950s depended on these devices to breath after being paralyzed with this devastating virus.

This iron lung was donated to the CDC's Global Health Odyssey by the family of polio patient Mr. Barton Hebert of Covington, Louisiana, who'd used the device from the late 1950s until his death in 2003.

Image courtesy of the CDC, GHO, Mary Hilpertshauser

Second Rehabilitation Theory

Dr. Sahrman's second generation of rehabilitation methods addresses people who have central nervous systems problems. A prime example of a central nervous system challenge is a stroke. A stroke occurs when the blood supply to part of the brain is blocked. When the blood supply is blocked, the brain does not receive the oxygen and glucose needed for the cells to function. This can lead to cell death. You often hear of people who have had a stroke losing their ability to talk or move certain parts of their bodies. This is a result of the damage to the brain from lack of oxygen and glucose.

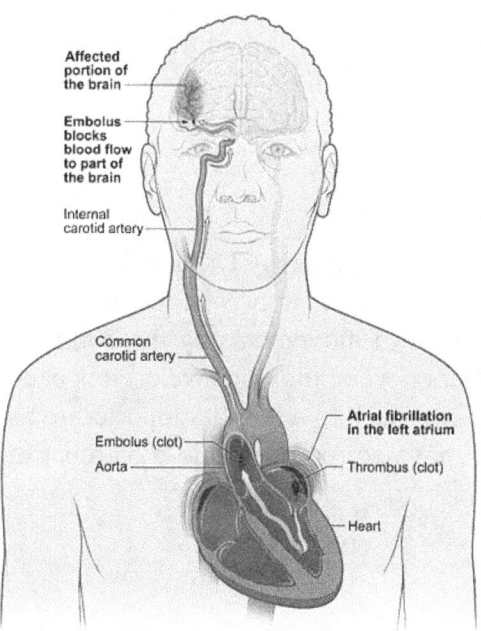

The illustration shows how a stroke can occur during atrial fibrillation. If a clot (thrombus) forms in the left atrium of the heart, a piece of it can dislodge and travel to an artery in the brain, blocking blood flow through the artery. The lack of blood flow to the portion of the brain fed by the artery causes a stroke. Image courtesy National Heart Lung and Blood Institute of the National Institutes of Health.

One thing that happens after a central nervous system challenge is that the muscles contract in a spasm. Spasticity is the constant contraction of the muscles caused by neurological problems. Since spasticity is controlled by the brain, and the brain is not working right after a CNS challenge, standard muscle strength testing does not work for assessing the patient. The muscle may, in fact be healthy, but is just not being controlled properly by the brain. There is still no standard of practice for assessing the muscles of patients with central nervous system problems. The brain is a complex organ. It is not well-understood by researchers or doctors. As imaging technology and other medical tools become more effective, doctors are better able to understand the relationship between damage to the CNS and muscle movement. As researchers and physicians learn more about this relationship, they will develop new techniques and tools for assessing and treating CNS challenges, as well as to maintain muscle health during recovery.

Third Rehabilitation Theory

This theory of rehabilitation introduces a muscle classification system based on strength and pain measures. Dr. James Cyriax championed this approach, which has allowed athletes to receive better treatment than they did in the past. In this approach, muscles are assessed based on whether a movement is strong or weak, as well as whether it is painful or non-painful. This approach takes into account the unique characteristics of each joint and its surrounding tissues. It was no longer necessary to simply limit the movement of the injured joint or muscle. The people treating the injury were able to develop treatment programs that take into account the unique nature of the injury, resulting in a much better treatment program for the athlete.

Fourth Rehabilitation Theory

The fourth rehabilitation theory identified by Dr. Sahrmann is a movement-based approach to treating injury. The movement-based approach includes basic anatomy and physiology, as well as neurological control of movements by the brain. Remember that we naturally take the path of least resistance when moving. We do this even if it may result in another injury down the road. This approach to rehabilitation focuses as much on ensuring that the brain is telling the body to move correctly as it does on repairing the actual injury.

Summary

Rehabilitation theory has changed significantly over the past several decades. Dr. Shirley Sahrmann has been a driving force behind these changes. She developed her first theory of rehabilitation based on her observations of muscle movement in polio patients. This led her to understand that muscle must heal fully before beginning strengthening exercises. The second theory addressed the different needs of a patient who had experience a central nervous system challenge, such as a stroke. The muscles may be healthy, but not receiving the signal to move in these patients. The third theory, which was supported by Dr. James Cyriax, resulted in a new way to test muscles for strength and pain. This led to improvements in rehabilitation programs. Finally the fourth theory, which is a movement-based approach to treating injury, involves treatment of both the injury and the way the brain tells the body to move.

Concept Reinforcement

1. Describe the concept of rehabilitation.

2. What did Dr. Sahrmann observe in polio patients?

3. Explain how the fourth rehabilitation theory incorporates everything Dr. Sahrmann already knew about rehabilitation.

Section 1.5 – Range of Motion

Section Objective

- Describe range of motion and discuss the different factors that can affect it (flexibility, mobility and stability)

Range of Motion

Range of motion is the ability of a joint to move and is an isolated measure of movement that can occur at a joint. Range of motion is tested on three planes of movement. A plane of movement is the direction in which the joint moves. There are three primary planes of movement: sagittal, frontal, and transverse.

Plane of Movement	Type of Movement
Sagittal	Horizontal – body cut into right and left.
Frontal (Coronal)	Anterior-posterior movement. Front-back movement. Body cut into front and back.
Transverse	Movement around a vertical axis, such as moving the head left or right. Body cut into top and bottom.

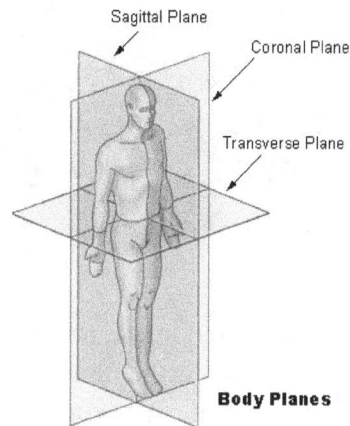

Image courtesy of cancer.gov

Range of motion is affected by three primary factors: flexibility, mobility and stability.

Flexibility

There are different types of flexibility: dynamic, static-active, and static-passive.

Dynamic flexibility is the ability of the muscles to move a joint through its full range of motion. Static-active flexibility is the ability to hold a position without using any external supports. For example, raising your leg in the air and holding it there for some period of time.

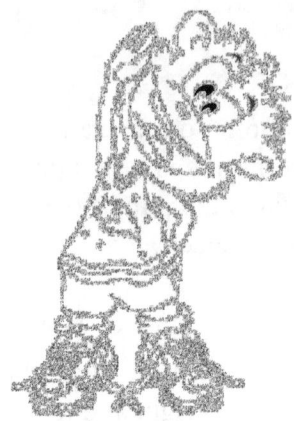

Slurp stretching
Image courtesy of US Department of Agriculture, Food and Nutrition Service

Static-passive flexibility is the ability to hold a position, using your weight or some type of support. An example is doing the splits or stretching on a ballet barre.

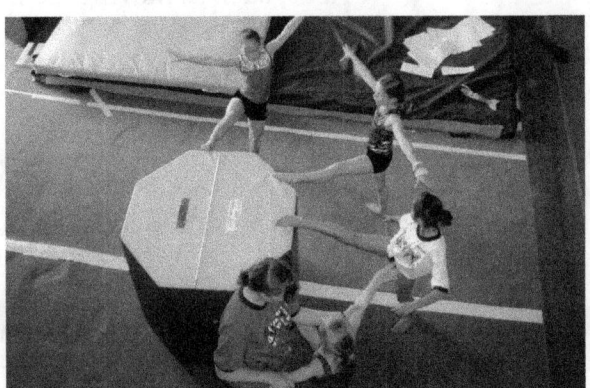

Girls stretching legs during a gymnastic training
Image courtesy of Rick McCharles

Dynamic flexibility is what we are interested in when talking about range of motion. When a person has limited range of motion, it means that the joint is unable to move as much as it should because of some sort of injury. In a healthy knee, the leg should extend straight out and be able to fold back until the heel touches the buttocks.

When a joint does not move fully and easily in its normal manner it is considered to have a limited range of motion. Motion may be limited by a mechanical problem within the joint, swelling of tissue around the joint, spasticity of the muscles, pain or disease.

Flexibility is the result of the muscle and connective tissues working together. As a muscle lengthens, the connective tissue stretches and becomes taut. If the connective tissue has lost its ability to stretch with the muscle, the joint will have limited range of motion.

It is also possible for a muscle to have too much dynamic flexibility. If the muscles become too flexible, the joint loses stability. Muscles will only stretch to their maximum length. Stretching beyond that simply causes the ligaments to stretch and the tendons to be strained. Both of these conditions make an athlete more prone to injury. In fact, a ligament will tear when it is stretched more than 6% of its normal length.

Mobility and Stability

Mobility and stability are related concepts. Mobility is the ability of a joint to move through a range of motion. Stability is the ability of a joint to support the body while it is moving. The Joint-by-Joint theory says that the joints in the body alternate between stable and mobile, which allows us to move as we need to. If a joint does not move properly, the faulty movement causes stress on the next joint, which can cause injury.

All joints have to move. Some have a much broader range of motion than others. The knee and elbow joints move forward and back. If you try to move them sideways, you will probably hurt yourself. The ankle, hip and shoulder joints, however, can move in many directions. This is what allows you to rotate your arm around your shoulder, sit crosslegged on the floor, and rotate your ankle in circles.

Summary

Range of motion is the ability of a joint to move as it is supposed to move. A limited range of motion is typically the result of a problem within or around the joint. It may be the results of tissue swelling, a functional problem within the joint, spasticity of the muscles, injury, or disease. Range of motion is affected by flexibility, mobility and stability. Flexibility is the range of movement in a joint. There are three types of flexibility: dynamic, static-active, and static-passive. Mobility and stability are related concepts. All joints are mobile – they are able to move. Joints may also be stable or mobile. A stable joint, such as the knee, typically has a range of motion limited to one plane. A healthy mobile joint, however, is able to move on all three planes easily. Problems in a mobile joint can cause problems in a stable joint and vice versa. This is because the force from a movement has to go somewhere. If the joint designed to absorb the force is not able to do so, the force moves up to the next joint, which is probably not able to absorb the force properly.

Concept Reinforcement

1. Define range of motion.

2. List the three planes of movement.

3. Explain how flexibility can enhance or limit mobility.

Section 1.6 – Muscle Stiffness

Section Objective

- List the four factors that contribute to stiffness in muscle tissues

What Is Muscle Stiffness?

Stiffness is the relative tension of the muscle. Stiffness is created by a muscle when it moves. Stiffness can be a positive or a negative sensation. Muscle stiffness may be associated with the joint. We want some joints to be stiff and others to be less stiff. The joints we want to be stiff are the joints that are stable according to the joint-by-joint theory. For example, the knee should be stable joint. The muscles surrounding the joint help provide the stiffness the joint needs to be healthy.

There are four factors that affect muscle stiffness: flexibility, muscle force capability, thixotropy, and extreme hypertrophy. We will address these one at a time.

Flexibility

There are three components of flexibility, which is the range of motion in a joint. Range of motion may be normal, limited or extended.

Dynamic flexibility is the ability of the muscles to move a joint through its full range of motion.

Static-active flexibility is the ability to hold a position without using any external supports. For example, raising your leg in the air and holding it there for some period of time.

Static-passive flexibility is the ability to hold a position, using your weight or some type of support. An example is doing the splits or stretching on a ballet barre.

> **Factors that Affect Muscle Stiffness:**
>
> Flexibility – the ability of a joint to move through its full range of motion.
>
> Muscle force capability: the force that a muscle is able to generate through movement.
>
> Thixotropy: reduced flexibility resulting from extended immobility.
>
> Extreme hypertrophy: Overdevelopment of muscles.

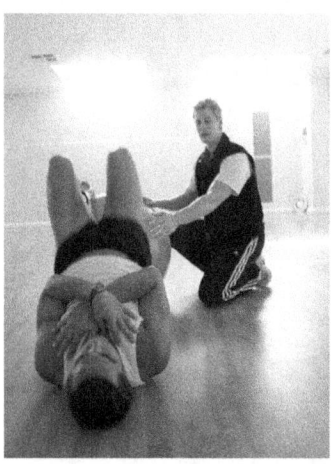

A person stretching

A muscle that is too tight limits a joint's range of motion, or ability to move through its full range of possible motions. Muscles that are too loose also cause joint problems. The muscles should work with the tendons and ligaments to support a joint properly. If the muscles are too loose, they do not provide enough support, which then strains the ligaments and tendons. This may lead to joint problems.

Muscle Force Capability

Muscle force capability is the ability of muscle to generate force when it contracts. Think about the force you can generate when you flex your bicep. Muscle contraction is measured using the **sarcomere**, the distance between two Z-bands in the muscle.

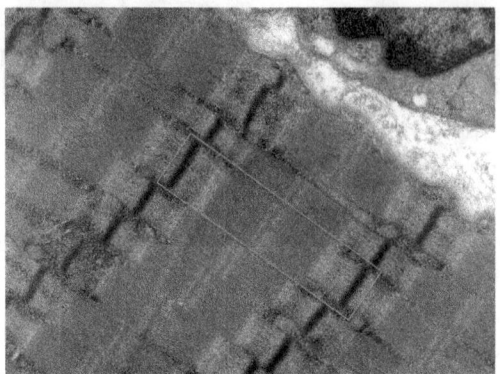

Transmission electron microscope image of a thin section cut through an area of human skeletal muscle tissue. The image of the muscle sarcomeres shows a distinct banding pattern: the darker bands are called A bands(the A band includes a lighter central zone, called the H band), and the lighter bands are called I bands. Each I band is bisected by a dark line called the Z-line). The red box outlines a sarcomere.

Image courtesy of Louisa Howard

The **sliding filament theory** describes how muscles generate force. The sarcomere is made of two types of muscle fiber: thin (actin) and thick (myosin). The sliding filament theory describes how thin and thick muscle fibers interact to generate force. Thin and thick muscle fibers slide past one another forming bridges. Maximum muscle force is achieved when the thin and thick muscle fibers interact as much as possible, forming the maximum number of bridges. Short muscles and muscles that are too long are not able to generate the maximum amount of force.

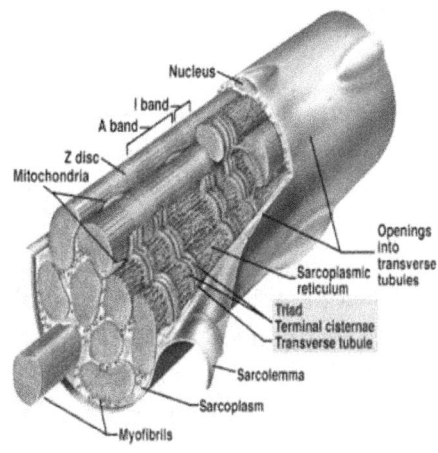

A graphic showing the sliding filament theory

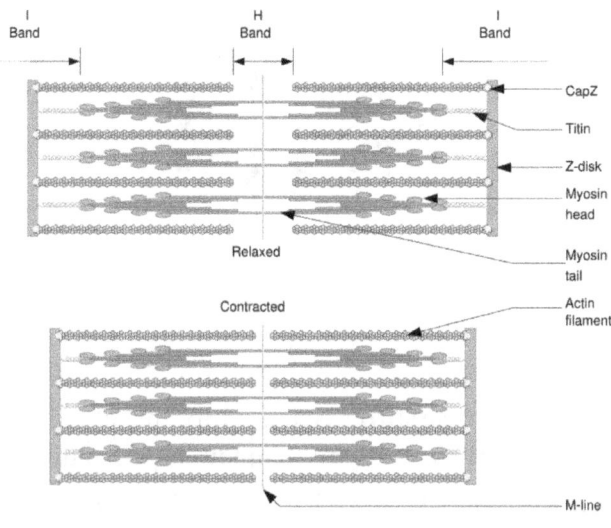

Muscle contraction

The force-length relationship describes the relationship between muscle length and the force generated by the muscle. As muscles contract, they get shorter. As they get shorter, they generate more force. This is true to the point where the muscles generate maximum force. The point of maximum force is different than the point of maximum contraction. Think again about doing a bicep curl. There is a certain point at which you generate maximum force, or ability to lift the weight. Once you get past that point, the force generated by the muscle movement decreases. Try doing a bicep curl and see if you can determine the point at which you reach maximum muscle force capability.

Thixotropy

Thixotropy describes muscle that has tightened after being immobilized for a long time. Muscles that are not able to move because they have been in a cast for long time, for example, lose their flexibility and ability to move easily. This condition can be corrected by following a well-designed stretching routine that coaxes the muscle into regaining lost flexibility and strength. Muscle that is not used atrophies, or wastes away, because it is not used. This is one reason that physical therapy is so important to patients who are bedridden for a long time or who have lost their ability to move because of paralysis or coma. Simply moving the muscles helps maintain flexibility and strength.

Hypertrophy

Extreme hypertrophy is overdevelopment of muscles. Think of the body builders who are bulky. Their muscles are hypertrophied because of all the body-building they do. Hypertrophy is actually a result of an increase in the size of individual muscle cells. As muscle cells grow, they increase the lean muscle mass of the person and increase how much the person is able to lift. Extreme muscular hypertrophy reduces flexibility, in part because of the sheer bulk of the muscle mass. It gets in the way of movement.

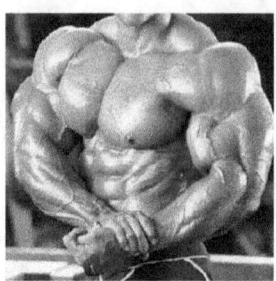

Extreme hypertrophy of muscle in a bodybuilder

Summary

There are four components of muscle stiffness: flexibility, muscle force capability, thixotropy and hypertrophy. Muscle flexibility is key to maintaining strength and the ability to move properly. Muscles that are too tight limit range of motion in a joint, just as muscles that are too loose can result in damage to the joint in the form of tendon or ligament tears. Muscle flexibility is important to maintaining healthy movement patterns and affects the ability of the muscle to generate force, or the ability to move weight. Muscle force capability is the ability of the muscle to generate force. The sliding filament theory describes how the thick and thin muscle filaments slide over one another to create bridges that generate force. Thixotropy is the tightening of immobilized muscle. Movement is necessary for flexibility, so muscles that do not move become tight, limiting range of motion and muscle force capability. Extreme hypertrophy is the overdevelopment of muscles, which can also limit flexibility, due in part to the bulk of the muscle mass limiting movement.

Concept Reinforcement

1. Define muscle stiffness.

2. Explain muscle force capability.

3. Describe the difference between thixotropy and hypertrophy.

Section 1.7 – Heart Rate

Section Objective

- Define resting heart rate, maximum heart rate, and training heart rate and discuss how each one is calculated

Heart Rate

Heart rate is measured by counting the number of times the heart beats in a minute. Three different types of heart rates are important in measuring fitness levels. These are resting heart rate, maximum heart rate and training heart rate. You measure your heart rate by taking your pulse. You can take your pulse anywhere on your body that you can feel it. The most common places are on the thumb side of the wrist (radial pulse); the inside of the upper thigh (femoral pulse), between the first and second toes (dorsal pedal pulse) and the front sides of the neck (carotid pulse). It is important to use only your index and middle fingers when taking your pulse. If you use your thumb, which is another place you can feel your pulse, you are likely to get an incorrect reading.

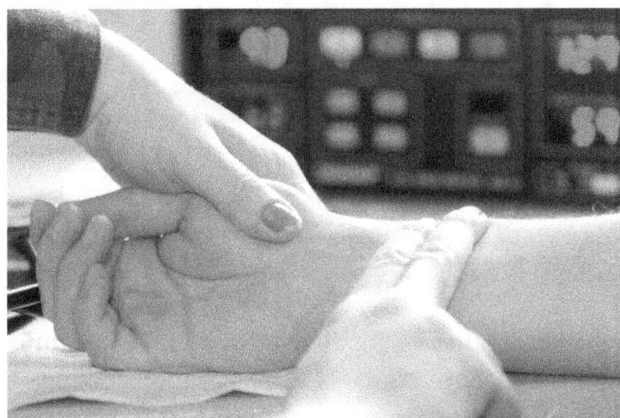

ROYAL AIR FORCE MILDENHALL, England — Airman 1st Class Stephanie Ambler checks the pulse of Capt. Derek Ferland to verify the accuracy on the automatic blood pressure machine during a blood drive here April 13. Airman Ambler is with the 48th Medical Support Squadron and Captain Ferland is with the 100th Civil Engineer Squadron.

U.S. Air Force photo by Staff Sgt. Jeanette Copeland

Resting Heart Rate

Resting heart rate is the rate your heart beats in a minute when you are at rest. The resting heart rate is measured in the morning immediately after waking up and before getting out of bed. Some experts recommend averaging the resting heart rate taken over three days to get the most accurate resting heart rate. This removes variability that could be introduced by a dream or the stress of waking up late.

Maximum Heart Rate

The maximum heart rate is the fastest your heart can beat. Maximum heart rate is difficult to measure. A standard method for estimating maximum heart rate is to subtract age from 220. This gives an estimate of heart rate, but studies have shown a 7-11 beat per minute error compared with other methods of estimating MaxHR. Stress tests are the most accurate way to measure maximum heart rate. A stress test is usually done on a treadmill that can increase in speed and incline. MaxHR is established when the person gives up and cannot go any longer, can't keep up with the treadmill, or when the heart rate levels off (plateaus). There are several ways of calculating MaxHR, each of which has different levels of accuracy.

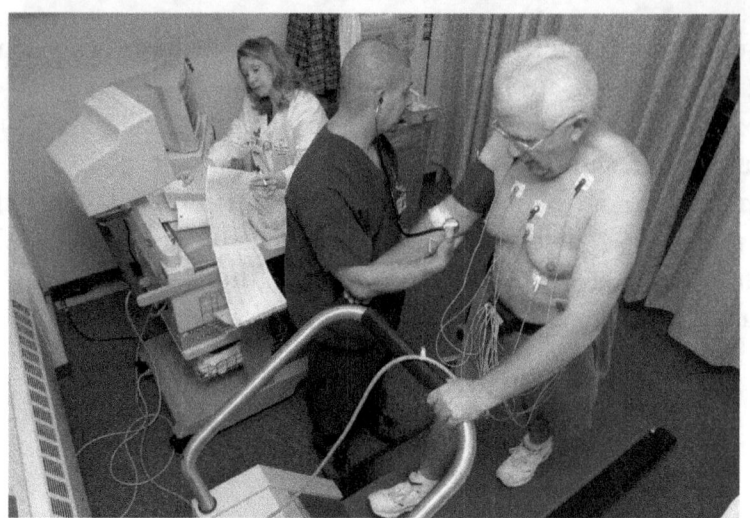

A patient undergoing a stress test

Training Heart Rate

Training heart rate is the heart rate you should achieve while in training. Training heart rate for short bursts of high intensity exercise is different than for lower intensity endurance exercise. The target heart rate (training heart rate) for high intensity exercise of short duration is 80-90% of maximum heart rate. Lower target heart rates of 60-70% are effective for promoting weight loss. A target heart rate of 70-80% of MaxHR will improve aerobic power.

Another way to determine your training level is to use the rating of perceived exertion scale. This scale was developed by Gunner Borg in 1973 and has been validated by several studies since then. The rating of perceived exertion (RPE) scale can also be used to approximate your training heart rate. Simply add a 0 to the Borg Scale to figure out your target heart rate. Your workout should have a rating of perceived exertion that falls in the green area.

\multicolumn{4}{c}{**Rating of Perceived Exertion Borg RPE Scale**}			
Scale	Intensity	Breathing Scale	Distance Scale
6	No exertion		
7	Very, Very light	Can sing full songs	Could continue all day
8			Could continue 4-6 hours
9	Very light	Can sing partial verses	Could continue 3-4 hours
10			Could continue 2-3 hours
11	Fairly light	Can talk in full sentences	Could continue 1-2 hours
12			Could continue 45-60 min.
13	Somewhat hard	Can talk in short sentences	Could continue 30-45 min.
14			
15	Hard	Breathing hard, thinking clearly	Could continue 15-20 min.
16			Could continue 10-15 min.
17	Very Hard	Breakaway ventilation*	Could continue 5-10 min.
18			Could continue 2-5 min.
19	Very, very hard		Could continue 1-2 min.
20	Maximum exertion		Could continue < 1 min.

*Breakaway ventilation is very rapid, deep breathing bordering on anaerobic effort and exhaustion. If you get to this point, you should lower your exertion level.

Summary

Heart rate is simply the number of times your heart beats in a given time frame and is usually measured in beats per minute. Three heart rates are important in sports medicine. Resting heart rate is your heart rate at rest and is usually measured before you get out of bed in the morning. Maximum heart rate, or MaxHR, is the fastest your heart can possibly beat. This heart rate is difficult to estimate. The standard tool equation for estimating maximum heart rate is 220 – age. Studies have shown that this equation results in 7-11% error in heart rate. A stress test is a more precise way to measure maximum heart rate. A stress test is done under the supervision of a physician or other qualified person. A stress test requires the subject to work as hard as they can until they cannot do any more or their heart rate plateaus. Finally, the training (or target) heart rate is the heart rate you want to achieve during your workout. One method of determining target heart rate is to use a percentage of your estimated MaxHR. The percent is determined by the type of workout you are doing. Another way is to use the rating of perceived exertion (RPE) scale, in which the athlete rates the difficulty based on perceived exertion. Target heart rate is often the RPE Scale number multiplied by 10.

Concept Reinforcement

1. What is the definition of heart rate?

2. List the three heart rates and what they represent.

3. Describe the Rating of Perceived Exertion scale.

Section 1.8 – Body Mass Index

Section Objective

- Define body mass index (BMI), describe how it is calculated and discuss the limitations of BMI calculations

Body Mass Index (BMI)

Body mass index is a measure of an individual's body mass in weight and in relationship to their stature (height). It is a measure of lean body mass and fat body mass. The calculation for body mass is simple. Weight in kilograms (kg) is divided by height in meters squared.

For example, the BMI calculation for someone who is 2 meters (6 ½ feet) tall and weighs 100 kilograms (220.46 pounds) is $100 \div 2^2$, or $100 \div 4$, which results in a BMI measure of 25.

BMI may also be calculated using pounds and feet/inches. The formula for this calculation is: BMI=(weight in pounds x 703) ÷ height in inches squared. Using our example above, the calculation looks like this:

$$BMI = (220.46 \times 703) \div 78^2 = 154{,}983.38 \div 6{,}084 = 25.47$$

The results are close, as you can see, but not exactly the same.

Other ways to calculate body composition.

There are other ways to calculate body fat, some of which are more reliable than BMI and some of which are less reliable. These include the waist-hip ratio, the pinch test, the bioelectrical impedance test, the immersion test, and the bod pod.

The **waist-hip ratio** is simple to calculate. It is simply a ratio of your waist measurement to your hip measurement. This measure gives you an idea of how much fat is stored in the abdomen. Abdominal fat increases the risk of heart disease. In general, women should have a ratio of 0.8 or lower and men a ratio of 1.0 or lower. The lowest healthy ratio is not known. In order to calculate the waist-hip ratio, simply divide your waist measurement (taken at the narrowest part of your waist) and your hip measurement (taken at the widest part of your hips). For example, a woman with a waist measurement of 34 and a hip measurement of 42 will have a waist-hip ratio of 0.81. This is the upper range of the healthy waist-hip ratio for women, but would be low for a man.

The **pinch test** is not a very reliable way to measure body mass index because so much depends upon the skill level and precision of the person performing the test. It uses calipers to measure folds of skin and fat in different places on the body (back of arm, abdomen, etc.). These measure are then averaged to get an estimate of body mass index.

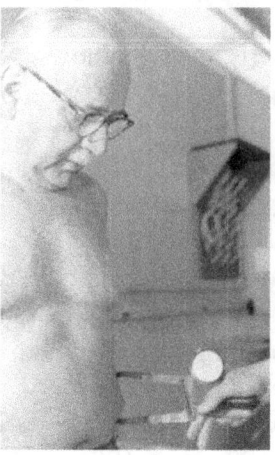

A man having a pinch test performed
Image courtesy of the National Institutes of Health

The **bioelectrical impedance test** is performed by running a radiofrequency pulse through the body to measure its water content. This method is more accurate than the pinch test, but can be skewed by exercise and liquid, which can decrease or increase the water content of the body.

The **immersion test** is the gold standard of body fat measurement. This is a difficult test to do because it requires the subject to expel all air from the lungs before being dunked into a pool of water so the water displaced by the subject can be measured. This process is done six times and the results averaged. This is an uncomfortable test for the subject. The results, however, are accurate within 1 percent.

The **bod pod** is another way to assess body mass index using displacement. This technique requires the subject to sit in an egg-shaped chamber for 20 seconds. The chamber measures air displacement. The air displacement and weight are used to calculate relative fat. This method gives better results for those who are densely muscled than the BMI calculation.

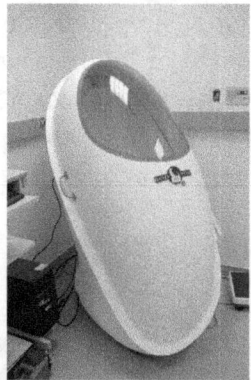

The Bod Pod
Image Courtesy of the National Institutes of Health

Body mass index measures do not take into account the mass of an individual that has more bone or muscle weight than fat weight. A short, very muscular person will probably have a BMI that is high even though he has far more muscle weight than the average person of that height does. This is a problem for many athletes, such as power lifters, who have more lean body mass than most people.

What is a healthy BMI?

The chart below shows the general height and weight measures associated with being underweight, normal range, overweight, and obese. The table uses both metric and English measures for weight and height.

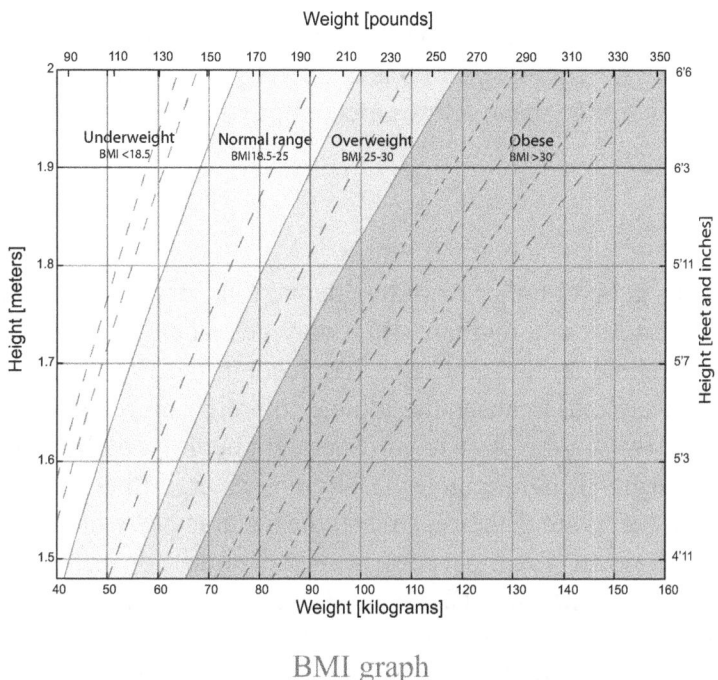

BMI graph

BMI is used to determine whether people are at a healthy body weight. Certain BMI measures are too low, which means the person is probably underweight, and others are too high, which means the person is probably overweight or obese. Both ends of the spectrum are associated with an increased risk of illness or death. A person whose BMI is too low may develop health conditions that are just as deadly as those developed by people whose BMI is too high. Look at the weight/height chart above to see where you fall. Think about whether the classification you fall into is an accurate representation of your fitness level.

The health risks associated with a high body mass index are:

- Type-2 diabetes
- Coronary heart disease and stroke
- Metabolic syndrome
- Certain types of cancer
- Pregnancy complications
- Sleep apnea
- Osteoarthritis
- Gallbladder disease
- Fatty liver disease

Low BMI (under 17) usually indicates protein-energy malnutrition or the effects of wasting or a disease process, such as cancer. Protein-energy malnutrition can usually be addressed by correcting diet, however low BMI because of wasting or a disease process cannot usually be corrected.

Athletes who are underweight often have other problems. Women with an extremely low BMI often experience amenorrhea. Amenorrhea occurs when the menstrual cycle shuts down because the body does not have enough fat to support a normal pregnancy. Being underweight may also indicate an eating disorder or other health problem that should be evaluated by a doctor.

Athletes with a high BMI may or may not have a high percentage of body fat. Athletes tend to be more densely muscled than non-athletes, which results in athletes weighing more than a non-athletes of the same general build. Remember that muscle weighs more than fat. Why is this important? A light person who is not fit may have a high percent body fat while a heavy person who is fit may have a low percent body fat.

Summary

Body mass index is a general indicator of health and risk for disease. BMI is a measure of the ratio of body fat and lean body mass. BMI may be calculated using height and weight measures, but this technique does not take into account the extra muscle an athlete may have. This extra muscle mass causes the athlete to weigh more. Remember that muscle weighs more than fat by volume. As a result, a straight height-weight ratio does not always work well for measuring BMI in athletes. There are several other ways to measure body mass index. The least accurate is the pinch test, the accuracy of which is highly dependent on the skill of the technician. The most accurate is the immersion test or the bod pod, which both use displacement to measure BMI. The BMI is calculated using a volume/weight calculation. Low and high BMIs both have health risks associated with them. Low BMI may indicate malnutrition, anorexia, wasting, or weight loss resulting from disease. High BMI may indicate that a person is overweight, but it can be deceptive in athletes, who tend to carry more muscle than non-athletes do.

Concept Reinforcement

1. State the definition of body mass index

2. List three ways to calculate BMI and state whether they are accurate or not.

3. Explain the limitations of BMI calculations.

Section 1.9 – The Five-Level Model of Body Composition

Section Objective

- Describe the five levels of body composition

Body Composition

Drs. Zi-Mian Wang, Richard N. Pierson Jr, and Steven B. Hemsfield developed the five-level model of body composition in the early 1990s. They published their findings in the American Journal of Clinical Nutrition in 1992. The purpose of this model is to provide a different framework for the study of body composition. The new technologies available for doing this research made it necessary to develop a new way of organizing the information about each level, as well as the interactions between levels.

The **five levels of body composition** are the atomic level, molecular level, cellular level, tissue-system level, and whole body level.

Level 1: Atomic Level

The first level of body composition is the atomic level. Atoms are the smallest form of an element. Elements are the matter that makes everything on the planet. Elements form all living and non-living things. Gold, for example, is an element. Oxygen is also an element. Elements fall into three primary groups, as shown in the periodic table of the elements. These groups of metals, metalloids, and non-metals.

Group →	1	2	3	4	5	6	7	8	9	10	11	12	13	14	15	16	17	18
↓ Period																		
1	1 H																	2 He
2	3 Li	4 Be											5 B	6 C	7 N	8 O	9 F	10 Ne
3	11 Na	12 Mg											13 Al	14 Si	15 P	16 S	17 Cl	18 Ar
4	19 K	20 Ca	21 Sc	22 Ti	23 V	24 Cr	25 Mn	26 Fe	27 Co	28 Ni	29 Cu	30 Zn	31 Ga	32 Ge	33 As	34 Se	35 Br	36 Kr
5	37 Rb	38 Sr	39 Y	40 Zr	41 Nb	42 Mo	43 Tc	44 Ru	45 Rh	46 Pd	47 Ag	48 Cd	49 In	50 Sn	51 Sb	52 Te	53 I	54 Xe
6	55 Cs	56 Ba		72 Hf	73 Ta	74 W	75 Re	76 Os	77 Ir	78 Pt	79 Au	80 Hg	81 Tl	82 Pb	83 Bi	84 Po	85 At	86 Rn
7	87 Fr	88 Ra		104 Rf	105 Db	106 Sg	107 Bh	108 Hs	109 Mt	110 Ds	111 Rg	112 Uub	113 Uut	114 Uuq	115 Uup	116 Uuh	117 Uus	118 Uuo

Lanthanides		57 La	58 Ce	59 Pr	60 Nd	61 Pm	62 Sm	63 Eu	64 Gd	65 Tb	66 Dy	67 Ho	68 Er	69 Tm	70 Yb	71 Lu
Actinides		89 Ac	90 Th	91 Pa	92 U	93 Np	94 Pu	95 Am	96 Cm	97 Bk	98 Cf	99 Es	100 Fm	101 Md	102 No	103 Lr

The Periodic Table of the Elements

All the tissues in the body are made of atoms of the elements necessary for us to live. The key elements are oxygen, carbon, hydrogen, nitrogen, and calcium. Other elements that occur in small amounts are phosphorus, sulfur, potassium, sodium, chlorine and magnesium.

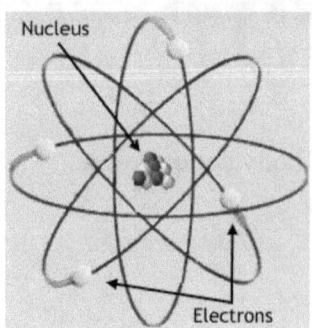

The percentages of the eleven principal elements found in an average man (70 kg) are:

- Oxygen   61.00%
- Carbon   23.00%
- Hydrogen   10.00%
- Nitrogen   2.60%
- Calcium   1.40%
- Phosphorus   0.83%
- Sulfur   0.20%
- Potassium   0.20%
- Sodium   0.14%
- Chlorine   0.14%
- Magnesium   0.027%

Level II: Molecular Level

Molecules are combinations of elements held together by bonds. The eleven principal elements shown above combine to form more than 100,000 different chemical compounds, all of which are found in the body. The key groups of molecules found in the body are water, protein, lipid, mineral and carbohydrate.

The percentages of each type of molecule are below. Again, these percentages are for an average man (70kg).

Water*

    Extracellular   26.00%

    Intracellular   34.00%

Lipid

> *Nonessential (fat)   17.00%*
>
> *Essential   2.1%*
>
> *Protein   15.00%*
>
> *Mineral   5.30%*

*Extracellular water is outside the cell and intracellular water is within the cell.

Water is the most common molecule in the body. Water makes up about 60% of body weight in an average man.

Proteins include all compounds that contain nitrogen. These compounds include amino acids and more complex molecules called nucleoproteins, which occur in the nuclei of cells.

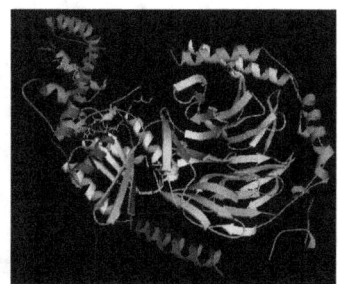

A protein image

Glyogen is the form in which the body stores glucose in the body. Glycogen is stored in the cytoplasm (the material inside a cell). It is usually found in the liver and skeletal muscle. Carbohydrates, on the other hand, is a much larger group of molecules that includes glycogen, glucose and other sugars, and complex carbohydrates that are part of cell membranes and receptors. They are also important parts of glycoprotein hormones and other chemicals.

Minerals are inorganic (compounds that do not contain carbon) compounds that contain both metal and nonmetal elements. The metal elements include calcium, sodium, potassium and other trace elements. Some of the key nonmetal elements are oxygen, phosphorus and chlorine. Minerals are typically divided into two categories, those found in the bone (osseous) and those found in the other tissues of the body (extraosseous).

Lipids are often thought to be the same as fats. Technically, lipids are different than fats. Lipids are groups of chemical compounds that cannot be dissolved in water (insoluble), but can be dissolved in organic solvents such as benzene or chloroform. There are about 50 different lipids in the human body, which are divided into 5 categories: simple lipids, compound lipids, steroids, fatty acids and terpenes. Lipids are also categorized as essential or non-essential based on their structure. Essential lipids are important for forming cell membranes. Non-essential lipids (body fat) provide insulation and store energy. In the average man, about 10% of lipids are non-essential and the rest are essential lipids.

Level III: Cellular Level

The compounds formed at the molecular level combine further to form the cells of the body. There are three main components at this level: the cell, extracellular fluids, and extracellular solids. Extracellular means outside the cell.

Cells have all the characteristics of life (metabolism, growth and reproduction). Metabolism is the conversion of food to energy. Growth is the process of becoming larger. Reproduction is the ability to have offspring, or in the case of cells, to make copies of themselves (replicate). Scientists have split cells into four categories: connective, epithelial (skin, organ tissue, etc.), nervous, and muscular.

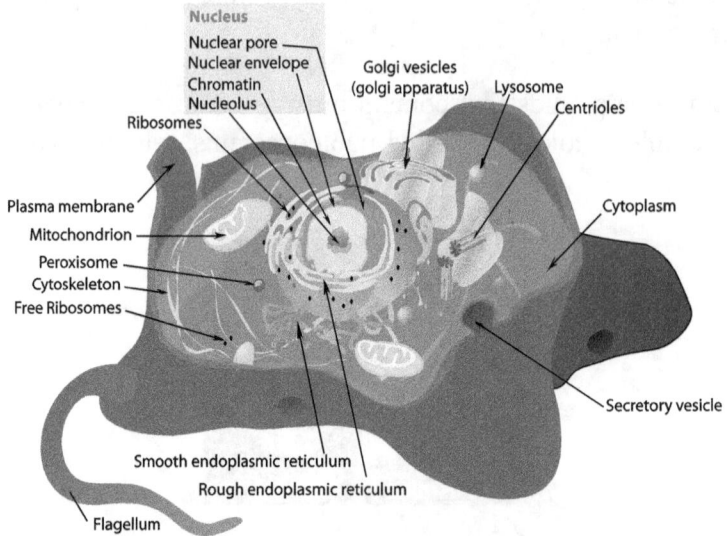

A cartoon of an animal cell. Each of the structures is composed of molecules.

Connective cells form the connective tissues of the bodies, such as tendons and ligaments. There are three groups of connective cells: loose, dense and specialized. Fat cells are an example of loose cells. Loose connective cells are located beneath the surface of the skin in an area called the dermis. Dense connective cells, fibroblasts, chondrocytes, and osteocytes are found in tendons, which have cells that are arranged in a regular pattern, the dermis of the skin, which has fibroblasts in irregularly organized collagen fibers, cartilage, and bone. Specialized connective cells are found in blood and bone cells.

Epithelial cells form the skin and the surfaces of organs. **Nerve** cells are found throughout the body and conduct messages from the brain to the body and vice versa. **Muscle** cells are divided into three categories: skeletal, smooth and cardiac. Skeletal muscles make up most of the muscle in the body and most of the weight in a human body.

Extracellular fluid is found outside the cells. This fluid allows for gas exchange, nutrient transfer, and excretion of metabolic waste. **Extracellular solids** include both organic and inorganic compounds. Collagen, reticular and elastic fibers are all extracellular solids. These solids are an important part of bone.

Level IV: Tissue/System Level

The cells of the body are composed of molecules, which are composed of atoms. Cells group together to form the tissues, organs and systems of the body.

Tissues contain cells that are similar to one another in appearance, function and origin in the embryo. As with cells, tissues are organized into the four categories of connective, epithelial, nervous and muscular tissues. Bone, fat and muscle tissue account for about 75% of the weight of the average man.

Organs contain two or more types of tissues that form larger functional units. The kidneys, pancreas, liver, heart, blood vessels, brain, and skin are all examples of organs.

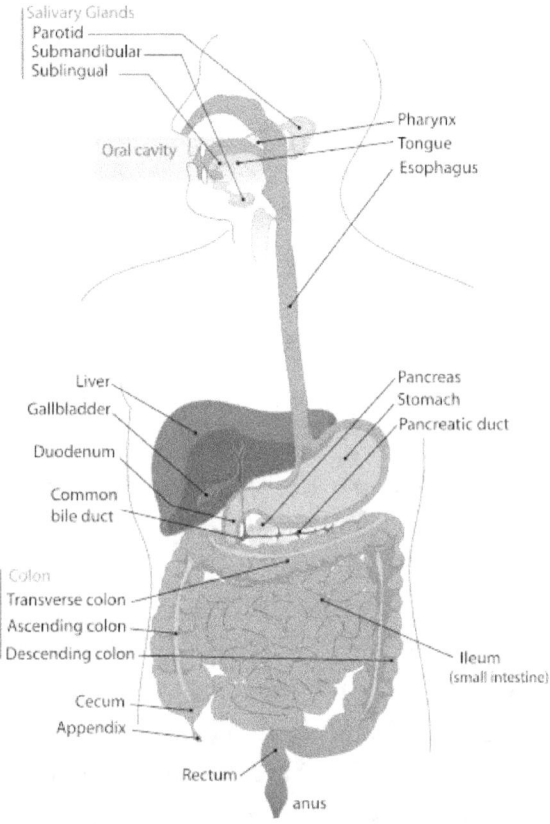

The Digestive System
Image courtesy of Miarian Ruiz Villarreal

Systems are made of several organs with related functions. The body has nine main organ systems: musculoskeletal, skin, nervous, circulatory, respiratory, digestive, urinary, endocrine and reproductive.

The list below shows the percent of body weight by system for a 70kg man.

Skeletal muscle   40.00%

Adipose tissue

    Subcutaneous   11.00%

    Visceral   7.10%

    Interstitial   1.40%

    Yellow Marrow   2.10%

Bone   7.10%

Blood   7.90%

Skin   3.70%

Liver   2.60%

Central Nervous System   2.00%

Gastrointestinal Tract   1.70%

Lung   1.40%

Level V: Whole body level

The whole body level of body composition includes the size, shape, and exterior and physical characteristics of the organism. The table below lists the primary characteristics of body composition.

Characteristic	How it is used to study body composition
Stature	Major indicator of body size and skeletal length
Segment lengths	The length of various segments of the body (arms legs, upper and lower arms and legs) are used to study body composition.
Body breadths	Used as a measure of body shape, skeletal mass and frame size. The wrist, elbow, knee, ankle and the biiliac (the widest measure between the iliac bones of the pelvis).
Circumferences	Used to understand bone density, fat mass, muscle mass, and energy stores. These are usually based on measures of the upper arm, waist and thigh.
Skinfold thickness	Estimation of fatness and the distribution of fat tissue. Measures are usually taken at the back of the arm, under the shoulder blade, the calf, and the abdomen. Skinfold thickness is used only for estimations. This is not a reliable way to assess body fat.
Body surface area	Body surface area is used to estimate basal metabolic rate and fat-free body mass.
Body volume	Used to estimate body size and calculate bone density.

Body weight	Used to screen patients for growth rates, obesity, and undernutrition.
Body mass index	A measure of total body fat.
Body density	A measure of the density of the body based on body weight and volume and is an indirect estimate of total body fat and fat-free body mass.

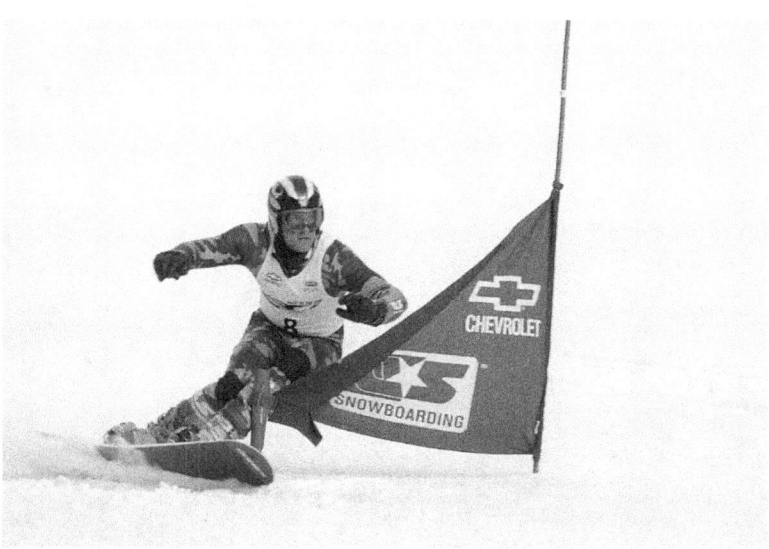

Spc. Ryan McDonald, a member of the U.S. Army World Class Athlete Program, slides around a gate on the slalom course at Copper Mountain, Colo., during the 2005 Continental Cup November 21 and 22.

Image courtesy US Army

Summary

As you may have figured out, each level of body composition is affected by changes in the other levels. Changes at the atomic, molecular, cell and tissue/organ levels have a measureable impact on the whole body. Nutrition affects how cells function, which affects how tissues and organ systems function. If a cell is not functioning properly, the entire organism may be affected. Muscles require a certain combination of nutrients to function at their maximum capacity. If the muscle cells do not receive these nutrients, they will not function properly. Similarly, if certain cells are damaged because of exposure to a toxic compound, it will affect how the overall organism functions. Most changes at the whole-body level are the result of changes in composition on one or more of the other four levels. This relationship allows researchers and sports medicine professionals to use measures of the whole body to estimate the composition of the other four levels of the body, as well as to adapt nutrition and workout programs to improve body composition.

Concept Reinforcement

1. List the five levels of body composition.

2. Describe how cells combine to form tissues.

3. Explain why the whole body level is useful in sports medicine.

Section 1.10 – Power, Speed and Agility

Section Objectives

- Define power, speed and agility and how each is measured

Power, Speed and Agility

Power is the ability to move a load. Every time you pick up an object, throw a ball, or swing a bat, you are using power to do something. Power is the ability to lift a load efficiently. In scientific terms, **power** is a function of strength and speed. Two athletes may be able to lift the same amount of weight, but the one who can move the weight faster demonstrates more power.

Speed is how long it takes to complete a task, such as lifting a heavy load or propelling a baseball across home base. **Agility** is related to speed. It is a function of speed and accuracy when doing a task that requires changing direction. Runners sprinting in a straight line demonstrate speed. A wide receiver demonstrates agility every time he changes direction to dodge a tackle.

Power, speed and agility are measured differently. Boxing combines all three. The punch has power and speed. Boxing also requires great agility and endurance.

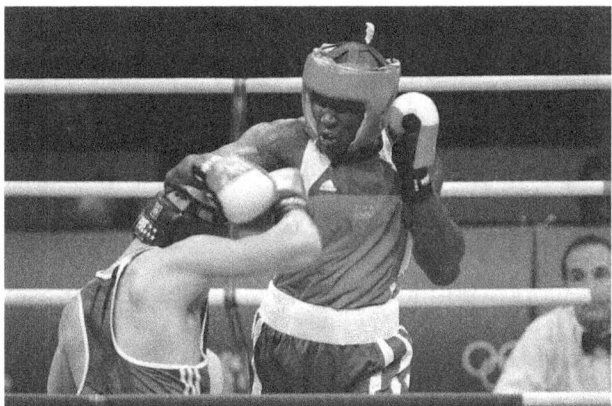

Straight on, medium shot of Olanda Anderson (Red) as he tries to land a punch against Rudolf Kraj, of the Czech Republic, in the Men's 81 Kilogram weight class at the 2000 Olympic games in Sydney, Australia, on September 24th, 2000. SSG Anderson is from the US Army's World Class Athlete Program, and he lost to Kraj by one point, 12-13.

Measuring Power

Power is a test of how quickly an athlete can move a sub-maximal load. A sub-maximal load is any load that is less than the maximum the athlete can move. Think of this in terms of weight lifting. If you are able to lift a weight more than once, the load is sub-maximal. "Maxing out" means that you can move the load once, which is a maximal load.

The calculation used to measure power is: $\text{Power} = \dfrac{\text{Force} \times \text{Distance}}{\text{Time}}$

Measuring power is a challenge because the technique and skill level of the athlete influence the power measured. Athletes require time and practice to become as efficient as possible in their movements. It probably will not be possible to get an accurate measure of power until the athlete masters the technique of the movement.

A general test of power that gets around the technique issue is the vertical jump test. The vertical jump test is a simple measurement of how high the athlete is able to jump. There are some easy-to-use measurement tools for measuring vertical jump. These include the Vertec and Just Jump mat. The Vertec is a pole with flags at different heights. The athlete's vertical jump is measured by the flags that he is able to tap with his hand. The Just Jump mat uses a pressure sensor to measure the time between take off and landing. It is then possible to calculate the height of the jump. Vertical jump is the easiest way to measure power.

Strong man competitions are power competitions. These competitions require the athletes to move a heavy weight a specific distance. The person who is able to accomplish this first shows the most power and also wins the competition. Competitors carry huge objects, pull vehicles, and do other feats of strength during these competitions.

Measuring Speed and Agility

The important thing to keep in mind when testing speed and agility is to use a test appropriate to the sport. For example, the speed of a baseball player can be tested with sprints that go in a straight line. The length around a baseball diamond is 120 yards, therefore a 100-yard sprint is a good measure of the player's speed. The speed of an athlete who plays American football is measured by how long it takes him to run the 40 yard dash. The sprinter who is a member of the 1,600 meter relay team will be assessed on how long it takes her to sprint 400 meters. Speed is measured in the amount of time it takes to move a specified distance. Sprint speeds are measured in seconds per distance covered. Usain Bolt from Jamaica set a new world 100-meter sprint record at the 2008 Summer Olympics when he ran the race in 9.69 seconds.

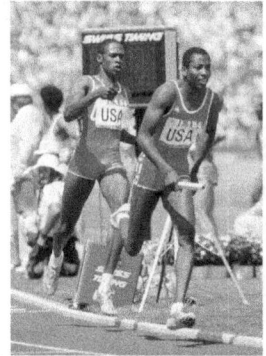

Second Lieutenant Alonzo Barbers (with baton), US Air Force, competes in a leg of the 4 x 400 meter relay at the 1984 Summer Olympics. Barbers won a gold medal in the event.
Image courtesy of: US Department of Defense. Photo by Ken Hackman, 14 August 1984

Agility is important in certain sports, such as tennis, soccer and American football. The **Pro Agility Drill** is a good tool for assessing agility. This drill is performed in a 10-yard space. The athlete starts the drill by straddling the middle line, then sprinting 5 yards in one direction, 10 yards in the opposite direction, and then 5 yards back to the middle. This drill measures the quickness of the athlete's stops and starts, as well as his use of mechanics to move efficiently. Sports that use this agility drill include football, baseball, volleyball, basketball, tennis, and any other sport that requires rapid directional changes.

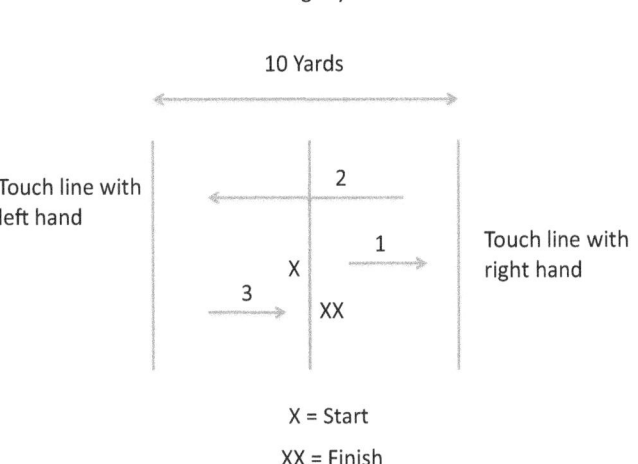

Teams use many other agility drills to ensure their athletes are as agile as possible. The drills used in football will probably be different than those used to train tennis athletes because the sports are fundamentally different.

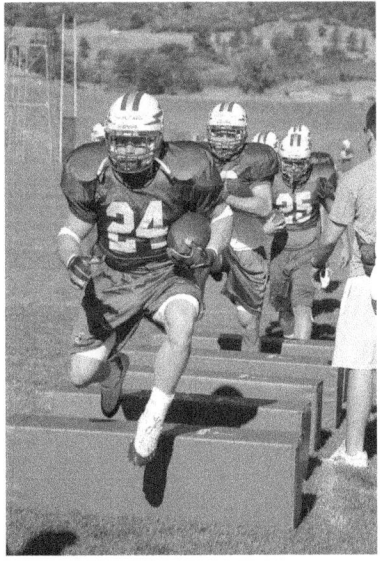

Falcons sophomore halfback Chad Smith leads fellow backs through an agility drill. Smith ran 34 times for 190 yards and one touchdown in the Falcons' triple-option rushing attack last season.
Image courtesy of U.S. Air Force/John Van Winkle

Summary

Power, speed and agility are three different aspects of movement. Power is the ability to move a sub-maximal load. Speed is the ability to move quickly from point a to point b. Agility is the ability to change directions quickly and efficiently while sprinting. Tests for power assess a combination of strength and speed. An athlete who can move a sub-maximal load more quickly than another athlete exhibits more power. Likewise, an athlete who is able to change direction quickly using efficient mechanics is more agile than one who does the same task less efficiently.

Concept Reinforcement

1. State the definition of power.

2. Explain the difference between speed and agility.

3. List one test each for power, speed and agility.

Section 1.11 – The Functional Movement Screen

Section Objectives

- Define the functional movement screen
- List the seven movements of the functional movement screen

The Functional Movement Screen

The functional movement screen (FMS) is a system developed by Gray Cook, Lee Burton and Keith Fields for evaluating the quality of a person's movement patterns. The FMS screens movement using seven basic movements. The functional movement screen is useful for screening a person's quality of movement. The FMS provides information that will help predict the person's chance of sustaining an injury, as well as whether the person has achieved optimum physical performance through a training program. This screening tool may be used on its own or as part of a more comprehensive screening, assessment and evaluation program.

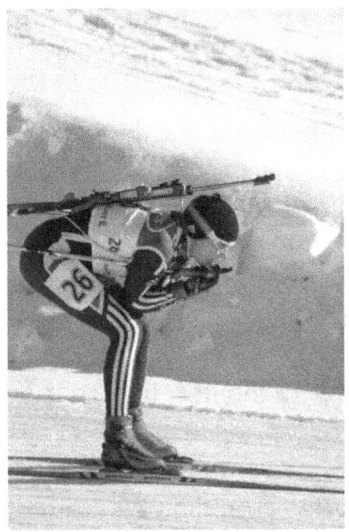

Army SPC Denise Teela participated in the Army World Class Athlete Program in the Women's Biathlon. In order for her to succeed in her sport, her movement needs to be healthy. The Functional Movement Screen is one tool that could be used to assess her movement patterns and develop a corrective program, if necessary.
Image courtesy of US Army.

The functional movement screen is based on how infants move as they develop. Newborns have the most primitive movement patterns that babies use to learn how to do more refined and complex movements. Infants go from lying on their backs and exploring their hands and feet to rolling. When babies learn to roll, they are learning to control how to move their bodies in a specific direction, eventually rolling over on their stomachs. Once babies are able to control their bodies enough to roll over, they begin to use their arms and legs to support their bodies. Once they have learned how to do this, they are able to crawl.

Eventually, the babies will learn how to stand and walk with assistance. As they learn to control their balance, babies are able to walk on their own. Walking turns into running, which can turn into even more complex movements as the baby grows and develops. Think about the control required to dance, play sports, or ride a bicycle. As babies learn how to walk, they also learn how to stand back up after they fall. This the point at which they have gained control of their bodies and how to balance their body weight.

Age	Motor Skills Developed
0-3 months	Head control Lifts head when lying facedown Beginning to learn to turn from side to back Kicking and stretching become more vigorous Grasp becomes stronger
4-6 months	Increased control of arms and legs Increased rocking on stomach, possibly rolling over May try to push themselves up or try to stand. Sit independently by 6 months. Hand-eye coordination improves.
7-9 months	Roll over in both directions, even when sleeping. Begin to scoot, rock back and forth, and crawl. May stand and furniture surf. Learn to move move things from one hand to another. Pick up objects with thumb and forefinger
10-12 months	Continue to develop ability to sit and move. Continue to develop ability to stand and move with support. May learn to walk.
1 year	Walk by 15 months, then run. Able to stop, squat and stand again. Able to sit down, climb stairs, dance with music, push and pull toys, and throw a ball overhead.

The functional component of the FMS refers to the functional aspects of movement. What is the most efficient way to use your body to do a vertical leap? There are functions that directly impact the quality of the vertical leap. There are other, less direct functions of the body that also impact the quality of the vertical leap because they improve the overall quality of movement. This means that direct and indirect training methods can improve the quality of movement. A direct training method to improve the vertical jump is practicing the vertical jump. An indirect training method is doing exercises that strengthen other parts of the body, such as exercises that strengthen the muscles of the hips and legs.

The functional pyramid includes three components of movement that are part of the functional movement screen. These include functional movement, functional performance, and functional skills.

The functional movement screen takes between six and twelve minutes to perform and consists of seven different movement patterns. The first step is to screen the patient for right/left asymmetries, or unbalanced movement on the right and left sides. Patients who have right/left asymmetries are referred to medical professionals for assessment and treatment.

For those patients who pass the first screen of the FMS, the next step is to have the patient perform the seven different movements of the functional movement screen. A few basic tools are needed to perform the FMS. You will need a 2x6 board, a 4-5' dowel or stick, a setup to make a hurdle, and a tape measure.

The seven movements of the FMS are scored on a scale of 0-3, with 0 being the lowest score and 3 being the highest.

Score	What it indicates
0	The movement is painful and the patient should be referred to a medical professional. This score is given for any movement that results in pain, regardless of whether the patient is able to perform the movement perfectly.
1	The patient is unable to perform the movement.
2	The patient is able to perform the movement, but has to compensate.
3	The person is able to perform the movement without compensating.

Movements are scored for each side of the body, so each movement of the functional movement screen will result in a score of 1-2, 1-3, 2-3, or 3-3. If the movement is asymmetrical (unbalanced from side to side), the asymmetry is the first thing that should be addressed in the training program because asymmetry is a leading indicator of the potential for injury.

The Seven Movements of the Functional Movement Screen

The Deep Squat

The deep squat is done using a symmetrical double stance, which means that your feet are planted just wider than shoulder width with the toes pointed straight forward. The dowel is pressed overhead and the patient squats as deeply as possible.

The Hurdle Step

The hurdle step is done using a symmetrical double stance, just as the deep squat above.

The dowel is on the shoulders in a back squat position and the patient steps over the hurdle at knee height.

The Inline Lunge

The inline lunge test requires the patient to hold the dowel on the shoulders while standing in the asymmetrical double stance, with one foot in front of the other. Drop to floor in split squat or lunge position with one knee on the ground.

Shoulder Mobility

The shoulder mobility test is performed by raising one arm, bending at the elbow, and attempt to reach down across the back. The palm should be facing the upper back. Lower the other arm behind the back and attempt to reach up with back of hand against the back. Try to bring the two hands together. Make fists with each hand with thumbs tucked in.

Active Straight Leg Raise

The patient lies on the floor with legs extended and together and toes pointed straight up. The patient raises one leg as far as possible.

Trunk stability pushup

The trunk stability pushup is performed on the floor. The patient places his hands on the floor near his forehead (near chin for women) and performs the "up" part of a push-up.

Rotary Stability

This test requires the patient to start out on hands and knees. The patient lifts the arm and leg on the same side, then brings the knee and elbow together.

FMS Screen	Form	Screens	Infant Movement Pattern	Adult Movement Pattern
Deep Squat	Double symmetric stance dowel pressed overhead deep squat	Ankle mobility Knee stability Hip mobility Core stability in the double symmetrical stance Torso mobility Shoulder blade stability Shoulder mobility	Baby getting up for the first time	Squatting Standing chair sitting against the wall Deadlifting

Hurdle Step	Double symmetric stance Dowel on shoulders Step over hurdle	Stability of supporting leg Mobility of stepping leg Core stability while in the one leg stance	Baby walking	Walking Going up and down steps Running Kicking
Inline Lunge	Assymetrical double stance Dowel held vertically behind back. Drop to floor in lunch or split squat position.	Ankle mobility Knee stability Hip mobility Core stability in the assymnetrical double stance Torso mobility	Baby not falling forward when walking	Stopping Changes of direction
Shoulder Mobility	Tuck thumbs into fists. Reach behind back with one arm reach down from overhead and the other reaching up from the waist. Try to touch fists together.	Torso mobility Shoulder blade stability Shoulder mobility	Baby reaching for objects Touching for exploration Sensory integration	Reaching Throwing Swinging implements.
Active Straight Leg Raise	Lie on back with legs extended and together Toes pointed up. Lift one leg as far as possible straight up.	Core stability Hip mobility	Baby reaching feet to explore the body	Hip flexibility Moving legs with trunk upright and stable Kicking
Trunk Stability Pushup	Lie on stomach with hands in push-up position at the forehead (males) or chin (females. Perform up part of push-up.	Core stability	Crawling and transitioning to standing	Pushing and pulling with arms while keeping the trunk stable (not moving with the arm movements)

Rotary Stability	On hands and knees, lift arm and leg (same side) from the floor. Bring knee and elbow together.	Core Stability	Rolling Crawling	Reaching to side Twisting safely

Summary

The Functional Movement Screen (FMS) is a way to screen the way a patient or athlete moves. The Functional Pyramid includes functional movement (bottom), functional performance (middle) and functional skills (top of the pyramid). The FMS rates movement on a scale of 0-3, with 0 meaning there is pain and the patient needs to go to the doctor to 3, which is good movement without pain or compensation. The assessment is done for each side of the body, so each movement will receive two scores – one for the left side and one for the right. The seven movements are the deep squat, inline lunge, shoulder mobility, hurdle step, rotary stability, trunk stability pushup, and active straight leg raise. Each movement assesses the mobility and stability of different parts of the body. Each movement also relates to both primitive infant movement and adult movement patterns.

Concept Reinforcement

1. Describe the Functional Movement Screen.

2. List the three components of the functional pyramid, from bottom to top.

3. List the seven movements in the Functional Movement Screen.

Section 1.12 – Stretching

Section Objectives

- List the four basic components of movement preparation (warm-up)
- List the four categories of stretching and discuss the characteristics of each

Movement Preparation

The warm-up is the first part of any workout. Warm-up exercises are important for preventing injuries as well as preparing to move more actively in the workout itself.

A well-designed warm-up meets four goals:

1. Increase tissue temperature
2. Increase muscle extensibility (ability to stretch)
3. Prepare the body to move in a single-leg stance
4. Prepare the central nervous system for higher levels of activity.

Your body goes through some specific changes during warm-up. As you begin to move and stretch, your tissue temperature and heart rate increase. The increased heart rate causes increased blood flow, which in turn results in increased total body temperature. One of the positive changes to your body during exercise is the movement of blood from the internal organs to the extremities (arms and legs). This movement of blood is important to maintaining good circulation in the hands and feet, as well as moving oxygen through the body.

Another result of increased blood flow and tissue temperature is that your muscles become more flexible. Another way of describing this is increased **extensibility**. Some of the standard exercises, such as the hamstring stretch and the butterfly stretch, are effective in increasing muscle extensibility. Stretching is more comfortable after you have warmed up your body for a few minutes by walking or doing some other form of movement. As we discussed, the increased blood flow resulting from movement makes the muscles more extensible, or flexible.

The Four Categories of Stretching

There are four generally accepted categories of stretching, which are active, static, passive, and dynamic. These four categories are combined to form four styles of stretching:

- passive static
- active static
- passive dynamic
- active dynamic

Passive stretching is done when the stretch is driven by an outside force. This outside force can be a person helping you stretch or a strap/rope that you use to apply the pressure you need to perform the stretch.

Active stretching is stretching that you perform without any outside help. You generate the force required to perform the stretch.

When you do a **static stretch**, you hold the stretch for some period of time before returning to the beginning position.

A **dynamic stretch**, on the other hand, means that you move from one stretch position to another without returning to your starting position.

How are these styles of stretching applied to a specific motion. We'll use bent-leg hip flexion as our example. In general, bent-leg hip flexion is bending your knee so your hip has to flex. This stretch can be done in a number of different ways.

Passive Static bent-leg hip flexion stretching is performed when lying on your back. You achieve your stretch when a person helps you stretch or you use a tool, such as a band or rope, to induce the stretch.

Active Static bent-leg hip flexion occurs when you stand up against a wall, and then kick the knee straight up toward the chest. The active static form of this stretch requires you to use your abdominal muscles and hip flexors to move the leg and hold it up.

Passive Dynamic bent-leg hip flexion stretches are done in the pushup plank position. In this stretch, one knee is forward with the foot flat on the floor near the hand on the same side. The pressure of the body on the foot provides the external force required to stretch the hip.

Active Dynamic bent-leg hip flexion stretches start in the pushup plank position, just like the passive dynamic version of the stretch. The primary difference is that the switch from one side to another is done continuously, so that you look like you are crawling.

Some research has shown that active dynamic stretching seems to be the most efficient in improving flexibility and performance after warm-up. The exaggerated patterns of movement improve the extensibility of the muscles, overall tissues temperature, and forces the body to prepare the body to perform the movements required during competition. Once you have warmed up, you are better able to be mobile, stable and aware of where your body is in space (proprioception), all of which are essential for competition.

Another benefit to active dynamic stretching is that the stretches are performed with enough intensity to take the joints through their entire ranges of motion, as well as being done quickly enough to increase heart rate. The increased heart rate ensures that the central nervous system is ready for the challenges of training and competition.

Concept Extension: Basic Stretching Routine

Neck Stretch

Tilt head to one side. Keep shoulders down. Place opposite hand on the side of the head and gently pull the head toward the shoulder. Hold for 10-30 seconds. Switch sides and repeat.

Calf Stretch

Stand facing wall with one foot forward and one back. Lean against the wall for 10-30 seconds, keeping feet parallel and rear heel on the floor. Switch legs and repeat.

Spinal Stretch

Sit in chair with back straight, feet on the floor with toes pointing up slightly. Lock fingers behind the head, with elbows out and chin down. Contract the abdominal muscles and twist the upper body to one side as far as possible. Repeat four times in that direction. The last time, rotate, hold and then lean forward with your elbow toward the floor. Return to seated position. Repeat on the other side.

Outer Thigh Stretch

Place left hand on wall to maintain balance. The arm and shoulder should be facing the wall. Place left foot behind and beyond the right foot. It looks like you are stepping sideways with your right foot in front of the left. Bend left ankle and lean into the wall. Hold 10-30 seconds then repeat on the other side.

Hip Stretch

Start on hands and knees. Bring one foot forward until the knee is directly over the ankle and the foot is pointing straight ahead. Lean forward into knee, lower the pelvis and the front of the hip toward the floor. Hold 10-30 seconds. Switch legs and repeat.

Butterfly Stretch

Sit on floor, bringing the soles of your feet together in front of you as close to your body as is comfortable. Your knees should be relaxed to the sides. Apply mild pressure to the legs to push the knees down slightly to increase the stretch. Hold for 5 seconds and repeat.

Thigh Stretch

Lie on stomach with legs together. Have a partner bend your lower leg until you feel a stretch in the front of your thigh. Repeat. Switch legs.

Crossover Stretch

Lie on your back. Bend one knee at a 90 degree angle and extend your arms out to the sides. Place your opposite hand on the bent knee and pull the knee over the other leg. Turn your head to look back toward the outstretched arm. Pull knee toward floor, being sure to keep your shoulders flat on the floor. Hold for 10-30 seconds and repeat on the other side.

Thigh Stretch

Lie on back. Place a band or rope loosely around the sole of one foot, holding one end in each hand. Lift the leg as high as possible toward the ceiling. Keeping your upper body on the floor, move your hands higher on the rope to enhance the stretch. Hold for two seconds and release. Repeats 8-10 times, then switch to the other leg.

Lumbar Stretch

Lie on back. Place one hand behind each knee and gently pull your knees toward your chest. Be sure to keep your lower back on the floor. Hold for 10-30 seconds, relax and repeat.

Summary

Stretching is an important part of every exercise program and should be done every time you work out. The four goals of a warm-up program are to increase tissue temperature, increase muscle extensibility (ability to stretch), prepare the body to move in a single-leg stance, and prepare the central nervous system for higher levels of activity. Stretching is divided into four categories: active, passive, dynamic, and static. These four categories are combined to describe four types of stretches. These are passive-static, active-static, passive-dynamic, and active-dynamic. Active dynamic stretching seems to be the most effective after the body has warmed up through some other form of movement, such as walking or jumping.

Concept Reinforcement

1. List the four goals of a well-designed warm-up program.

2. List the four categories of stretches.

3. Explain the difference between passive-static stretching and passive dynamic stretching.

Section 1.13 – Corrective Exercise Program

Section Objectives

- Describe how a corrective exercise program is utilized to improve faulty movement patterns

What is a Corrective Exercise Program?

A corrective exercise program is used to help patients who are in rehabilitation. The patient may be in rehabilitation because of an injury or illness. A corrective exercise program is basically a way to correct poor movement and help a patient who is recovering from an injury. Patients in rehabilitation for an injury perform corrective exercises in the early phases of treatment. The corrective exercise program often evolves into a warm-up program. The reason for this is because the exercises from the corrective exercise program, if continuously used in warm-up programs, can help minimize the risk of injury in the future.

A corrective exercise program focuses on the weak links of the patient, often based on a screening tool like the Functional Movement Screen. A corrective exercise program also focuses on the movement changes required for an individual to minimize the patient's susceptibility to injuries. It can also help reduce the amount of compensation the patient makes in his movement that could lead to re-injury or new injuries.

A good corrective exercise program has the same goals as a good warm-up program. The patient should have increased tissue temperature, increased muscle extensibility, be preparing to move the body on one leg, and have the brain prepared for the higher level activities of training and competition.

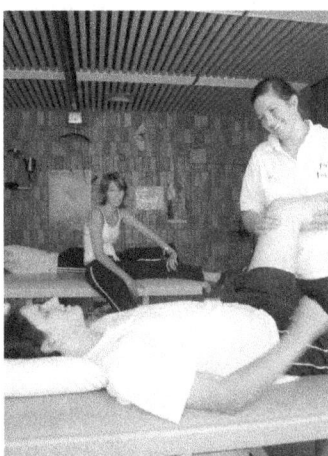

Physical Therapy Session

A corrective exercise program should also include screening for faulty movement patterns and a plan for correcting the faulty movement patterns. The Functional Movement Screen

(FMS) is a well-accepted methodology that identifies weakness or imbalance in movement. Other screening methodologies use gait, the overhead squat, or the single-leg squat as assessment tools. All screening methodologies are used to assess what needs correction. The assessment findings are used to develop a correctional exercise program for any faults that are found.

Many individuals with movement dysfunctions continue to train even though they have lost mobility in specific joints. Some individuals may not even know they have a movement dysfunction, so continue to train and cause more damage and dysfunction. Strength training, which is often considered an essential part of a training program, will cause more faulty movement patterns and joint dysfunctions.

Corrective exercise programs are used for more than treating and preventing sports injuries. These programs are also used to treat movement dysfunction related to poor work place ergonomics, injuries from accidents, and other things that can cause movement problems.

Concept Extension: A Sample Exercise Program to Help Relieve Neck Pain

The following set of exercises is used by a trainer to keep his neck and shoulders mobile and pain free.

Levator Stretch

Sit on a bench or chair. Reach behind your back at waist level with one hand. Tilt your head forward and point your nose toward your opposite hip. Place your other hand on your head and apply gentle pressure forward. Hold for 30 seconds or more. Switch sides and repeat.

Thoracic Mobility

You will need a foam roller or two tennis balls taped together for this exercise. Place the roller under your mid back. Keep your hips down while rolling up and down 2-3 times. Move the roller higher (more toward the shoulder blades) and repeat. This is inappropriate for the lower back – do not use the roller under your lumbar spine.

Face Down Touch Down

Lie face down on a bench. Point your thumbs toward the ceiling and raise your arms above your head like you are signaling a touchdown. Repeat 10-15 times.

Wall Slide

Stand with your back touching a wall. Slide your arms up the wall as high as possible, while keeping your head, shoulders, hands and elbows in contact with the wall. Slide your arms back down, again maintaining contact.

I Give Ups

Raise your arms above your head and shrug your shoulders. Perform 10-15 repetitions.

Summary

A corrective exercise program is used to help a patient rehabilitate from an injury or surgery. A corrective exercise program is designed based on a screening of the patient, using the Functional Movement Screen or some other screening tool, to assess movement dysfunction. As the patient recovers from the injury or surgery that caused the joint dysfunction, the corrective action program becomes part of the warm-up program. These exercises are included in the warm-up program because they will continue to strengthen the injured joint and help prevent future injuries.

Concept Reinforcement

1. State the purpose of a corrective exercise program.

2. Explain why an assessment of movement is done before a corrective exercise program is designed.

3. Why is a corrective exercise program incorporated into the patient's warm-up routine?

Section 1.14 – Muscle Tissue Quality

Section Objective

- Describe the methods used to improve muscle tissue quality

Muscle Tissue Quality

Muscle tissue quality is defined as the amount of skeletal muscle strength per unit of muscle mass. Muscle tissue quality can be measured in a variety of ways, each of which results in slightly different ways of interpreting muscle tissue quality. It can be measured using the **1 rep max**, the maximum amount of weight you can lift one time, **muscle peak power**, the amount of work that the muscle can do in the shortest time possible, or **muscle peak torque**, the amount of rotational force the muscle can generate around a joint.

Factors Affecting Muscle Tissue Quality

Muscle consists of bundles of **muscle fibers**, individual muscle cells. Each muscle fiber contains numerous actin (The most abundant protein in a eukaryotic cell) and myosin (A family of motor proteins that moves actin) filaments, special proteins that can form crosslinks. When the two filaments form crosslinks, the heads on the myosin filaments bend, sliding the two filaments past one another. The heads detach, reposition themselves, and begin the process again. This ratchet-like sliding movement is how muscles contract. The muscle fibers actually become shorter but thicker. The number, frequency, and duration of neural signals to the muscle determine how many muscle fibers are activated, thus affecting how strongly the muscle contracts.

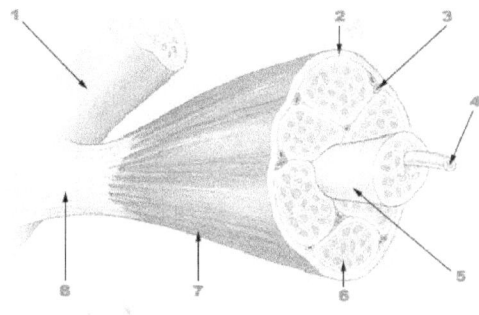

Skeletal muscle

1. Bone – structural tissue
2. Perimysium – a sheath of connective tissue that contains groups of muscle fibers
3. Blood Vessel – a vessel that allows blood to move nutrients to cells and remove waste from cells
4. Muscle Fiber – muscle cells
5. Fascicle – a bundle of muscle fibers contained by the perimysium
6. Endomysium – sheath of connective tissue surrounding a muscle fiber
7. Epimysium – a sheath of connective tissue surrounding an entire muscle.
8. Tendon – a fibrous connective tissue that connects muscle to bone.

The force a muscle is capable of generating is directly proportional to the cross-sectional area (CSA) of the muscle. The larger the muscle, the greater the contractile force it can generate. Muscle tissue quality is a measurement of the ability of a muscle to achieve its potential given its size. High quality muscle tissue is capable of generating force because it contains more actin and myosin filaments and is more responsive to neural stimulation than poor quality muscle. As noted above, there are several ways to measure muscle tissue quality. However, regardless of how muscle tissue quality is measured, it can be affected by age, adiposity, and exercise.

Muscle tissue quality tends to decline with age. We tend to lose muscle mass as we age. This is called **sarcopenia**. This is interesting because we lose strength more quickly than we actually lose muscle mass. Part of this change is because more of the muscle is taken up by connective tissue and fatty deposits. This maintains some of the muscle cross-sectional area (which is directly related to its mass) while decreasing the amount of the muscle that is made up of contractile elements. Even though the muscle may be the same size, it has fewer actin and myosin filaments.

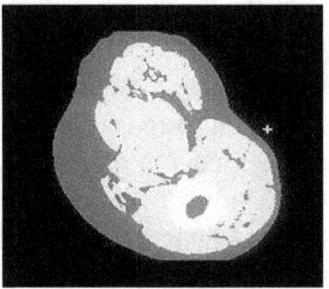

CT scan of a thigh muscle of a healthy young adult. The thigh bone is white. The muscle area (yellow) is not indicative of sarcopenia.

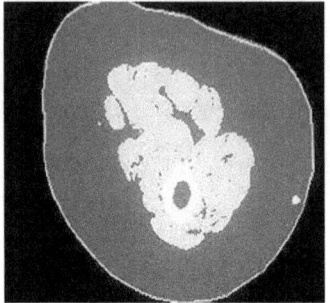

CT scan of a thigh muscle of a sedentary older adult. The thigh bone is white. The greatly reduced muscle area (yellow) indicates sarcopenia.

Adiposity, or fatness, affects muscle tissue quality because fatty deposits within and between the muscle fibers increase or maintain the cross-sectional area of the muscle without contributing to strength. The fat deposited between the large muscle fascicles is commonly called **seam fat** because it is found within the "seams" of the muscle. In the case of extremely obese people, there are actually fatty deposits within the muscle itself, **intramuscular fat**. In meat, this kind of fat is called marbling.

Finally, exercise, or the lack thereof, affects muscle tissue quality. Exercise affects the types of muscle fibers present in the muscle. **Type II fibers**, muscle fibers that use anaerobic metabolic pathways, are critical to maximum strength. **Type I fibers**, muscle fibers that use aerobic pathways, are more important for endurance. Lack of exercise allows muscle tissue to **atrophy**, or become both smaller and weaker.

Improving Muscle Tissue Quality

The best method to improve muscle quality is intensive resistance training using weights. Such training increases the cross-sectional area of type II fibers in the muscle, increases the number of muscle fibers activated during a movement, and increases **myofibrillar packing**, the number of actin and myosin filaments packed into a muscle cell. More actin and myosin filaments means more cross bridges can be formed, increasing muscular strength.

Proper diet to reduce excess adiposity will reduce the amount of fatty tissue deposited in the muscles. The result is that the cross-sectional area of the muscle will be occupied by tissue related to generating strength. A healthy diet includes plenty of fresh fruits and vegetables, lean proteins, and high quality carbohydrates. Highly processed foods, fatty meats, and low quality carbohydrates will have a negative effect on muscle quality.

Some people use androgenic steroids to improve muscle mass and strength. They may think these steroids also improve muscle quality, but this has not been proven. In fact, studies have shown that androgen therapy does NOT improve muscle quality. The proven ways to improve muscle quality are eating high quality food and engaging in strength-building exercises. Steroid use is not recommended for anyone whose body is still developing, and rarely for those who have finished growing.

Finally, although there is no way to reduce your age, exercise has been shown to return muscles to a more youthful profile and improve muscle tissue quality in elderly men and women. Simple exercises such as walking, yoga or weight lifting can make a large difference in muscle quality and the ability of elderly people to move.

Summary

Muscle mass, strength and quality are three separate concepts. Muscle mass simply refers to the amount of muscle a person has. Muscle strength is a measure of how much weight that muscle is able to move. Muscle quality is a measure of the muscle strength per unit of muscle mass. High quality muscle will have a higher ratio of muscle strength to muscle mass than low quality muscle. In part, this is because the high quality muscle has little fat tissue and has tightly packed, efficient muscle cells. Muscle with a lot of mass, even though it has a lot of strength, may not be as high quality as muscle with less mass. The muscle strength to muscle mass ratio indicates muscle quality. Consider this example. Two athletes are able to lift the same amount of weight when doing a bicep curl. One athlete is bulky and the other is not. It is likely that the athlete that is not bulky actually has higher quality muscle tissue. Muscle quality can be improved by engaging in intensive resistance training and eating a high quality diet. Exercise is important throughout life to maintain muscle quality and independence.

Concept Reinforcement

1. Explain how muscles contract.

2. What are the factors that affect muscle tissue quality?

3. How does adiposity decrease muscle tissue quality?

4. How does intensive resistance training with weights improve muscle tissue quality?

Section 1.15 – Nutritional Supplements

Section Objectives

- Define RDA and discuss why RDA may not provide sufficient vitamins and minerals to athletes and active individual

- Discuss how to objectively assess supplement claims

Why Are Nutritional Supplements of Interest in Sports Medicine?

The body requires certain nutrients to function at its best. Animals receive most of the nutrients they need from the food they eat. This is one reason it is important to eat a well-balanced diet of whole, nutritious foods. Food contains vitamins and minerals, which the body converts to energy. This energy is used to support all of the function of the body, including the involuntary (breathing, digestion, and other functions required to live) and voluntary (moving arms and legs, speaking, etc.).

How Does the Body Convert Vitamins and Minerals to Energy?

Enzymes are the proteins in the body and are responsible for changing the food we eat into the energy our bodies need to function. Enzymes are catalysts for the chemical reactions that convert food to energy. A catalyst is something that starts a process or allows it to occur more quickly. Think of starting a fire. The heat energy generated by striking the match catalyzes the flame, which is a chemical reaction between friction and the material on the head of the match. The chemical reaction generates heat energy (fire) and the waste product of charcoal or ash from the fire itself.

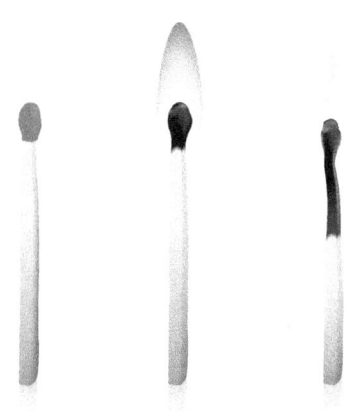

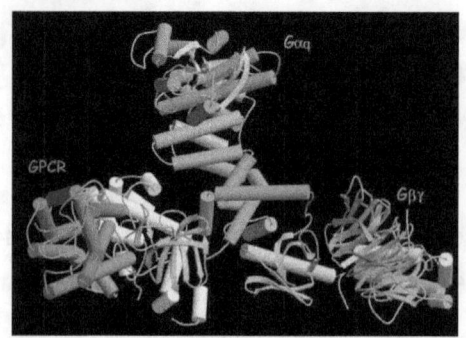

The structure of G proteins. These proteins exist in the cell and are molecular on/off switches for certain biological processes. These include the processes that control heart rate, blood pressure, glucose metabolism, as well as taste, smell and sight. The G proteins are activated by G-protein-coupled receptors (GPCRs), which reside in the cell membrane and react to specific external signals, such as light or adrenaline. In order for cells to adapt to changes in their environments out side the cells (extracellular environment), activated GPCRs must be rapidly desensitized. Desensitization is started by G-protein-coupled receptor kinases (GRKs), enzymes that phosphorylate (add phosphate groups to) the portions of activated GPCRs that project into the cell.
Image courtesy of the Advanced Light Source at the
Lawrence Berkeley National Laboratory.

Enzymes need co-enzymes to function. Coenzymes transport products between enzymes during the chemical reactions. Coenzymes are also called substrates, which means they are the substances acted on by enzymes. Vitamins and minerals are coenzymes in the human body.

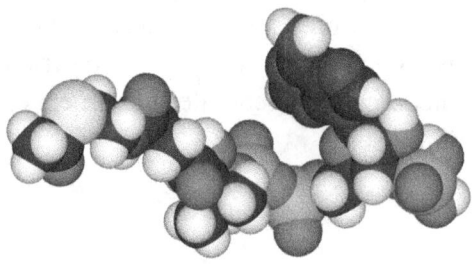

An acetyl coenzyme

Recommended Daily Allowance

Carbohydrates are the molecules of energy used by the body for healthy function. Enzymes catalyze (jump-start) conversion of carbohydrates that can be used by the body. If the body is missing certain vitamins and minerals because of a poor diet or physical problem, it may be necessary to take nutritional supplements to help the body convert carbohydrates into the energy we need to function.

The Recommended Daily Allowance (RDA) is a minimum level of vitamins and minerals required to maintain health. The US Department of Agriculture publishes these standards based on the average person in the country.

The following chart is adapted from the Food and Drug Administration's 1998 Food Labeling Guide.

Reference Values for Nutrition Labeling

(Based on a 2000 Calorie Intake; for Adults and Children 4 or More Years of Age)

NUTRIENT	UNIT OF MEASURE	DAILY VALUES
Total Fat	grams (g)	65
Saturated fatty acids	grams (g)	20
Cholesterol	milligrams (mg)	300
Sodium	milligrams (mg)	2400
Potassium	milligrams (mg)	3500
Total carbohydrate	grams (g)	300
Fiber	grams (g)	25
Protein	grams (g)	50
Vitamin A	International Unit (IU)	5000
Vitamin C	milligrams (mg)	60
Calcium	milligrams (mg)	1000
Iron	milligrams (mg)	18
Vitamin D	International Unit (IU)	400
Vitamin E	International Unit (IU)	30
Vitamin K	micrograms (µg)	80
Thiamin	milligrams (mg)	1.5
Riboflavin	milligrams (mg)	1.7
Niacin	milligrams (mg)	20
Vitamin B_6	milligrams (mg)	2
Folate	micrograms (µg)	400
Vitamin B_{12}	micrograms (µg)	6
Biotin	micrograms (µg)	300
Pantothenic acid	milligrams (mg)	10
Phosphorus	milligrams (mg)	1000
Iodine	micrograms (µg)	150
Magnesium	milligrams (mg)	400
Zinc	milligrams (mg)	15
Selenium	micrograms (µg)	70
Copper	milligrams (mg)	2
Manganese	milligrams (mg)	2
Chromium	micrograms (µg)	120
Molybdenum	micrograms (µg)	75
Chloride	milligrams (mg)	3400

Athletes and people who are active may require more than the RDA of vitamins and minerals because they are using more energy to perform their sports or other activities. The International Society of Sports Nutrition studies the nutritional requirements of athletes and published their findings for use by sports medicine professionals and others.

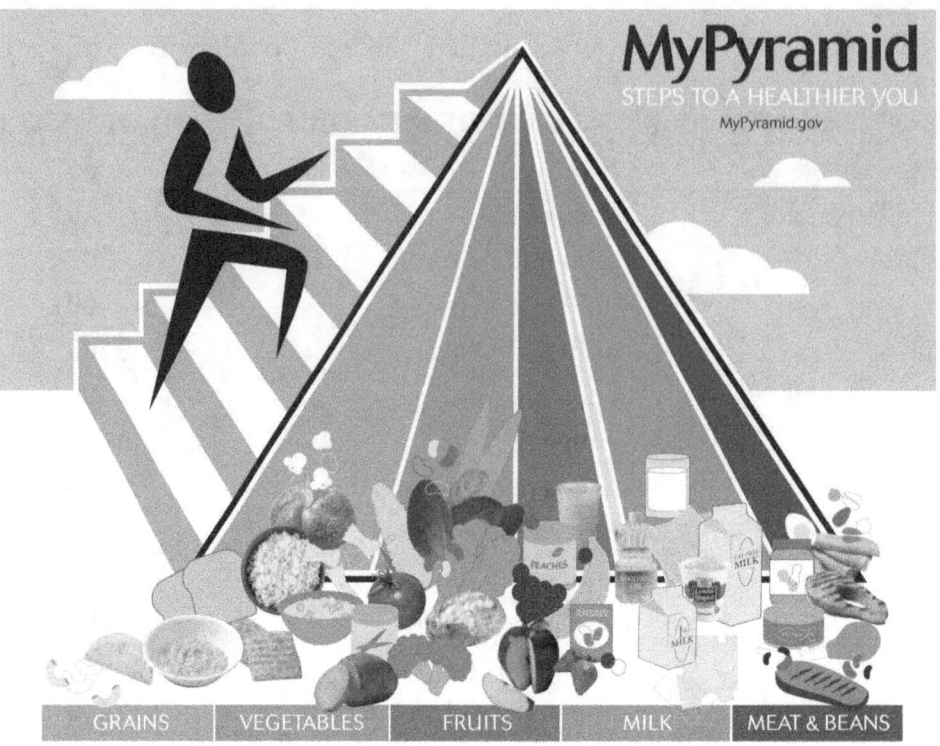

The food pyramid provides diet suggestions that will help you meet your nutritional needs with the food you eat.
Image courtesy of the US Department of Agriculture

Another consideration when making food choices is the waste products from the chemical reactions the body uses to convert the food to energy. The more food we put into our bodies, the more chemical reactions are required to convert the excess carbohydrates, fats and proteins in the food to usable energy. Free-radicals are byproducts of the chemical reactions used to convert food to energy. A free radical is an atom that needs more electrons. Oxygen and hydrogen are common free radicals. The body creates antioxidants to bind with the free radicals, reducing their ability to cause damage to the tissues in the body. The more food you eat, the more free radicals are released into your system. Your body may not be able to neutralize all of the free radicals, which is one time you may want to consider taking antioxidant supplements.

Rank	Food	Serving Size	Total Antioxidant Capacity per serving size
1	Small Red Bean	1/2 cup dried beans	13727
2	Wild blueberry	1 cup	13427
3	Red kidney bean	1/2 cup dried beans	13259
4	Pinto bean	1/2 cup	11864
5	Blueberry	1 cup cultivated berries	9019
6	Cranberry	1 cup whole berries	8983
7	Artichoke hearts	1 cup cooked	7904
8	Blackberry	1 cup	7701
9	Prune	1/2 cup	7291
10	Raspberry	1 cup	6058
11	Strawberry	1 cup	5938
12	Red Delicious apple	1	5900
13	Granny Smith	1	5381
14	Pecan	1 ounce	5095
15	Sweet cherry	1 cup	4873
16	Black plum	1	4844
17	Russet potato	1 cooked	4649
18	Black bean	1/2 cup dried beans	4181
19	Plum	1	4118
20	Gala apple	1	3903

Image courtesy of the US Department of Agriculture

Sports Supplements

Health and Health Education Act of 1994 requires a dietary supplement to supplement the diet in the form of a vitamin, mineral, herb, amino acid, or dietary substance noted as a part of the recommended total intake. A dietary supplement may be a combination of vitamins, herbs, minerals, amino acids, and other dietary substances.

The supplement must be in the form of a pill, capsule, tablet, powder, or liquid. It must be labeled as a dietary supplement and not as a food. The US Food and Drug Administration (FDA) does not regulate supplements unless sufficient complaints have been filed with them about a particular supplement. This is very different than the role they take in regulating and testing medications. All medications must be tested and approved by the FDA before they can be released for use by the public.

Scientific studies have shown that Americans tend to be deficient in certain vitamins and minerals. In a study of almost 500 individuals published in the Journal of the American College of Nutrition, researchers found that 30% of study participants were deficient in Vitamin C and 6% were severely deficient. Hyman and Liponis state in their book

"Ultraprevention" that the USDA found 37% of Americans are deficient in vitamin C, 70% in vitamin E, 75% in zinc, 40% in iron, and almost 100% in omega-3 fatty acids. These studies suggest that there is compelling evidence to consider taking a multivitamin to improve your health.

Remember, however, that it is important to understand fully the potential benefits and negative side effects of any supplement you choose to take. Be careful of assuming that "herbal" and "natural" automatically mean that a supplement is safe. Snake poison is natural, too! If you have questions, speak with an expert, such as a physician, pharmacist or nutritionist before you take anything.

Multivitamins

A multivitamin contains vitamins, minerals, or and other compounds that are considered essential to good health. Some multivitamins are for general use and others are specially formulated for particular groups of people.

Glucosamine and Chondroitin Sulfate

Glucosamine and chondroitin sulfate are two supplements that are commonly packaged together because of claims of improved efficacy when they are ingested together. These supplements have been studied and proven to help treat osteoarthritis, which athletes often develop as a result of injuries to the joints. Glucosamine is a sugar that occurs naturally in the body. Glucosamine is a component of glycosaminoglycans, which are the primary components of the hyaline cartilage of the bone. This cartilage covers the ends of the bones where they meet at the joints and provides cushioning between the ends of the bones. Hyaline cartilage wears down through the natural aging process, as well as because of overuse or misuse of the joint. When this occurs, osteoarthritis can develop. Chondroitin sulfate is another glycosaminoglycan and a major component of cartilage. Chondroitin sulfate fights compression in the joints, which is helpful in fighting osteoarthritis.

The recommended doses for glucosamine and chondroitin sulfate are 1500 mg (glucosamine) and 1200 mg (chondroitin).

Vitamin B12

Vitamin B12 is a water-soluble vitamin that is primarily involved in the creation and maintenance of brain and nerve cells and red blood cells. It also plays a role in DNA synthesis, which is the process of replicating DNA by combining the appropriate compounds. DNA is the genetic code for our bodies that holds all the information required for our bodies to form. It gives instruction in eye color, hair color and type, height, sex, and all the other physical characteristics of our bodies.

Vitamin B12 is typically found in meat, poultry, eggs, and milk products. Vegetarians sometimes need to supplement their diets with B12 in order to remain healthy.

Remember the role of B12 in the body – creation and maintenance of brain, nerve and red blood cells. It makes sense that the result of B12 deficiencies include fatigue, weakness and weight loss. A B12 deficiency may also result in parasthesia (tingling) and anaesthesia (numbness) in the extremities (hands and feet). These are peripheral nervous system changes. Central nervous system changes resulting from B12 deficiency include loss of balance and mental status changes. Interestingly, it seems that people over 50 years of age are less able to utilize natural forms of B12, but seem to be able to utilize the artifical forms of B12 found in nutritional supplements.

Here is another interesting point about B12. A study conducted at Oregon State University showed that even mildly decreased vitamin B12 levels can result in decreased performance capacity and ability to recover from exertion. In fact, some studies that suggest that the USDA RDA for vitamin B12 may be insufficient for athletes. Scientists have found that B12 products have an absorption rate of approximately 10 to 25% when taken in a capsule or tablet form. Because the tablet is taken with water or fruit juice, much of the liquid passes through the body in about 25 minutes. This means the stomach acids are left to degrade the solid form of B12, which reduces the amount absorbed into the body. When consuming certain commercial products that come in a liquid form, over 80% of the product is absorbed into the body. The form of the vitamin or mineral supplement is an important consideration when choosing a supplement.

Creatine

Creatine is an extremely popular sports supplement that gained popularity after the 1992 Olympics in Barcelona, Spain. Shortly after those Games, there were reports that some of the successful Olympians had used creatine supplements during training.

Creatine phosphate is substrate that is important for breaking down ATP (Adenosine Triphosphate). ATP is the body's preferred energy source. ATP is broken down to provide energy when we engage in highly anaerobic activities, which are those that do not require oxygen. Creatine phosphate is the source of energy for sprints, jumps, heavy lifting and other activities that do not require oxygen.

As ATP is broken down, one of the phosphate groups breaks off as a result of the chemical reaction. The phosphate then binds to creatine, which is delivered to muscle cells as energy. The scientific literature strongly supports that cells use up to 20% more creatine and creatine phosphate when performing anaerobic activities.

Creatine is typically packaged as a powder. The user mixes the powder with a liquid to ingest it. Creatine can also be ingested in capsule or tablet form. Taking creatine with a protein, amino acid, or carbohydrate has been shown to improve absorption into the body. Research has shown that creatine supplementation combined with a well-designed strength training program results in improved muscle cell performance, protein synthesis (the creation of new proteins, in this case of muscle fibers), satellite cell proliferation

(valuable as muscle cells incur damage during training, satellite cells can transfer cellular organelles to increase rate of muscle cell repair and hypertrophy), and clear improvements in strength and power.

Many other supplements are available, but we will not discuss them here. Supplements have various levels of safety and efficacy, so it is important to fully understand the potential benefits and risks to every supplement you take. It is also important to understand that people react differently to supplements. This may be based on their unique genetic profiles, age, or any number of other factors.

Summary

Dietary supplements may be useful in filling the gaps in nutrition that may result from your diet. In certain situations, it may not be possible to get all the nutrients you need from food alone. Nutritional supplements are useful for maximizing sports performance. It is important to understand the benefits and risks of the supplements before you decide to take them. The effects of supplements on performance and health have been studied for years and reports on the benefits of specific supplements are available. These studies may provide information on situations in which a supplement is useful, how different populations respond to the supplement, and other factors that should be considered before adding a particular supplement to your diet.

Concept Reinforcement

1. State the definition of RDA.

2. Explain why the RDA of a specific vitamin or mineral may not be sufficient for an athlete.

3. Describe how to assess the value of a supplement.

Unit Two

Section 2.1 – The Cardiovascular System   92

Section 2.2 – Measuring Cardiovascular Function   97

Section 2.3 – The Respiratory System   101

Section 2.4 – Lung Volume   103

Section 2.5 – The Skeletal System   107

Section 2.6 – Bone Tissue and Bone Health   111

Section 2.7 – The Stress-Strain Curve   115

Section 2.8 – Joints and Levers   119

Section 2.9 – The Muscular System   123

Section 2.10 – The Central Nervous System   127

Section 2.11 – The FIT Principle   131

Section 2.12 – Power, Strength, and Endurance   135

Section 2.13 – Interval Training: Aerobic and Anaerobic Conditioning   139

Section 2.14 – Sets and Repetitions   143

Section 2.15 – Thibaudeau's Six Training Programs   145

Section 2.1 – The Cardiovascular System

Section Objective

- Define the cardiovascular system and identify its main functions

The cardiovascular system

The **cardiovascular system** is comprised of the heart, the arteries that carry blood away from the heart, the veins that carry blood toward the heart, and the capillaries that allow blood to circulate through the tissues to provide them with oxygen and nutrients and carry away waste and carbon dioxide (CO_2). In the following discussion, we will examine the functions of the various segments of the cardiovascular system.

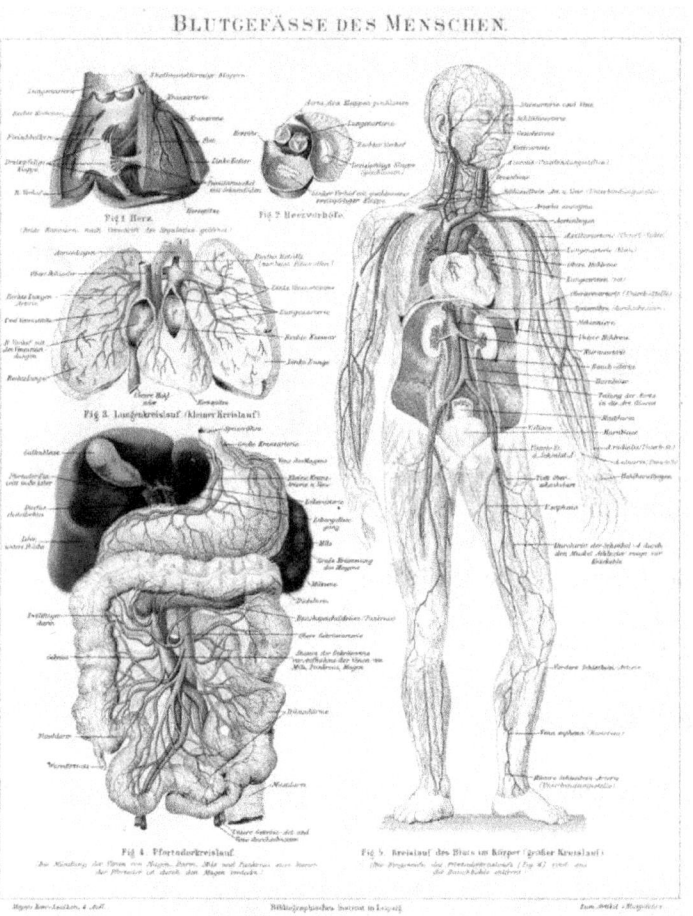

The Heart

The **heart** is the pump of the cardiovascular system. The average human heart beats about 72 times per minute. That is 2,838,240,000 beats over a 75 year lifetime! There are four chambers in the human heart, the right atrium, the left atrium, the right ventricle, and the left ventricle. The two atria fill with blood passively; there is no pumping action that forces blood into the atria. The atria force blood into the ventricles. The ventricles pump blood out of the heart. The right ventricle sends oxygen-depleted blood to the lungs, the left ventricle pumps **oxygenated**, or oxygen-rich, blood to the rest of the body. Valves separating the ventricles from the atria prevent blood from flowing backwards and prevent the mixing of deoxygenated and oxygenated blood.

The brain signals the heart to beat, stimulating the **sino-atrial node (SA node)**, a nerve complex located in the right atrium of the heart that coordinates the beating of the heart. The SA node passes the signal through the atrium to the **atrioventricular node (AV node)**. As the signal passes through the atrium, the atrium contracts to force blood into the ventricles. The AV node causes a slight delay to allow the ventricles to fill completely before it passes the signal to beat along special bundles of nervous tissue called **Purkinje (purr-KIN-gee) fibers**. The ventricle then contracts beginning at the bottom, pushing the blood up and out. As the ventricles contract, the atria relax and begin to fill again with blood.

Arteries

The **arteries** carry blood away from the heart. Many people make the mistake that the arteries carry oxygenated blood. While this is true in almost all cases, there are two very important arteries, the **pulmonary artery** and the **umbilical artery**, which do not. Instead, the pulmonary artery carries deoxygenated blood from the right ventricle to the lungs. The umbilical artery carries deoxygenated blood from the heart to the placenta, where it can exchange gasses and wastes with the mother.

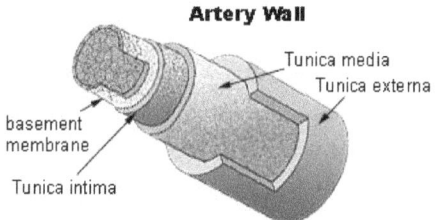

Arteries are elastic and capable of not only stretching to accommodate the pulse of blood as it exits the heart (this is the pulse you feel at your wrist or neck), but contracting to permit blood to flow or obstructing its passage. The arteries are partially responsible for blood pressure via their contractile property. They are also capable of redirecting blood flow where it is most needed. For example, under exercise conditions, blood is directed toward the muscles and away from the digestive system.

Veins

Veins carry blood toward the heart. Again, as is the case for arteries, people regularly make the mistake that veins carry deoxygenated blood. This is true in all cases except for the pulmonary vein and umbilical vein in the fetus, both of which carry oxygenated blood back to the heart. Veins exert little effect on blood pressure. Because they can generate so little pressure, the veins of the arms and legs contain valves to prevent blood from flowing backwards and pooling in the hands and feet. When the valves become damaged, blood can flow backwards and **varicose veins**, poor circulation, and **edema** (swelling and reddening of the tissue) result.

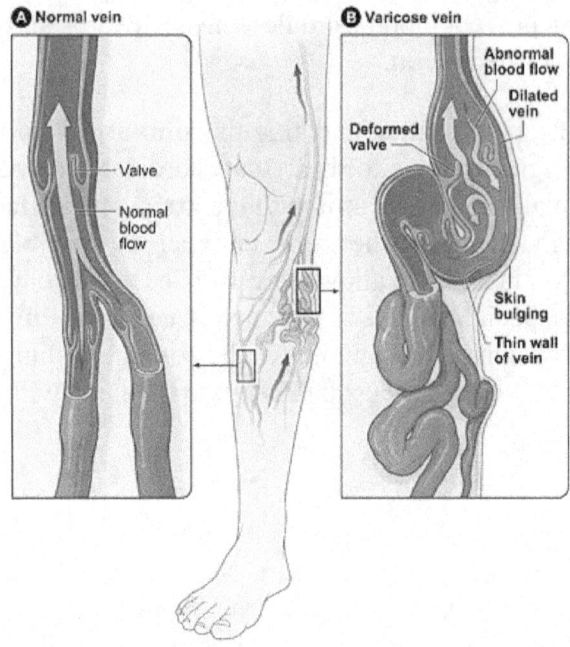

Capillaries

The arteries branch repeatedly as blood moves away from the heart toward the tissues. Finally, the arteries become so small that they are literally smaller in diameter than an **erythrocyte**, or red blood cell, which must bend and flex to pass through. These are **capillaries**, and they bring blood to within a few millimeters of the cells in the tissue. Capillaries are where oxygen is released into the tissues and CO_2 is picked up for return to the lungs. Nutrients are exchanged for metabolic waste products at the capillaries. Fluid passes out of the capillaries on the arterial side of the capillary bed and re-enters the capillaries on the venous side of the capillary bed.

Summary

The cardiovascular system is comprised of the heart, the arteries that carry blood away from the heart, the veins that carry blood toward the heart, and the capillaries that allow blood to circulate through the tissues to provide them with oxygen and nutrients and carry away waste and carbon dioxide (CO_2). Arteries are elastic and capable of stretching and contracting to permit blood to flow or obstructing its passage. Veins generate little pressure. Capillaries bring blood to within a few millimeters of the cells in the tissue. Capillaries are where oxygen is released into the tissues and CO_2 is picked up for return to the lungs. Nutrients are exchanged for metabolic waste products at the capillaries.

Concept Reinforcement

1. Describe the major parts of the cardiovascular system.

2. How do arteries and veins differ?

3. What are the functions of the capillaries?

Section 2.2 – Measuring Cardiovascular Function

Section Objective

- Describe three variables of measurement used to assess the functioning of the cardiovascular system

Cardiovascular System Function

The cardiovascular system must supply oxygen and nutrients to the body's tissues and remove carbon dioxide (CO_2) and metabolic waste products. To accomplish these tasks, the heart must effectively pump blood into the arterial system, the arteries must maintain enough pressure on the blood to push it through the vascular system and into the tissues, and the blood must enter the capillaries to **perfuse**, or pass a liquid through, the tissue. Medical professionals monitor the body's ability to accomplish these tasks using simple tests.

Cardiac Function

To measure **cardiac**, or heart, function, physicians use two easy-to-conduct tests, pulse and **electrocardiogram** (EKG). Your **pulse** is the number of times per minute your heart beats and is measured by **palpation**, *or* by touch or feeling, at the wrist. Physicians can determine not only the number of times the heart beats per minute, but the strength of the pulse, weak, thready, or strong. An EKG is a recording of the electrical activity of the heart as it beats. An abnormal EKG can tell the physician where the heart has a problem.

> An electrocardiogram is called an EKG instead of ECG to avoid confusion. ECG sounds very similar to EEG, which is an electroencephalogram, or a recording of the electrical activity of the brain.

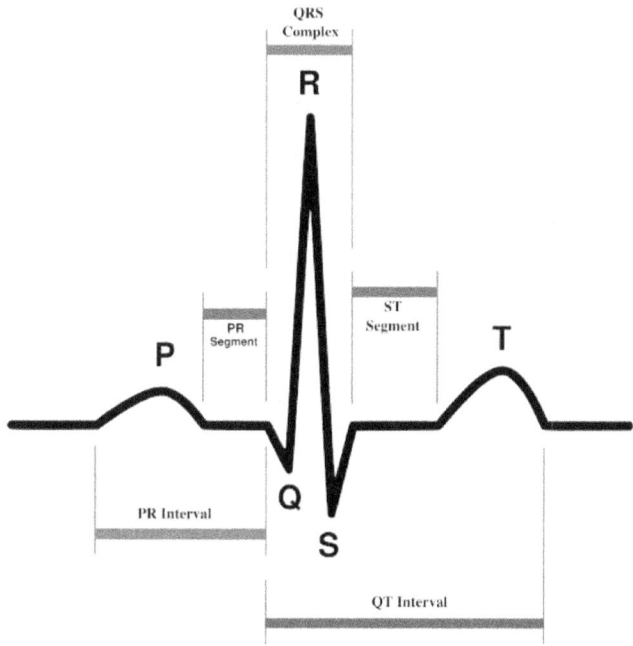

A schematic of an electrocardiogram of a normal heartbeat showing the entire process of a single beat.

Bradycardia (BRAY-dee-CAR-dee-uh), or excessively slow heartbeat, may indicate either a damaged **sino-atrial node (SA node)** or a damaged **atrioventricular node (AV node)**. The SA node is responsible for coordinating the beat of the heart and maintaining a normal heart rate. The AV node delays the transmission of the signal to beat to the ventricles momentarily to allow the atria to fill the ventricles with blood. Damage to either may result in a reduced heart rate. Bradycardia is usually classified as a heartbeat of less than 60 beats per minute (bpm). However, elite athletes may have heart rates below 60 bpm and still be healthy. This is because their hearts are very efficient at pumping blood. **Tachycardia** (TACK-ee-CAR-dee-uh) is an excessively fast heartbeat and depends upon age. Young children have much faster resting heart rates than adults. Beyond the age of 15, a heart rate of over 100 bpm is considered tachycardia. Tachycardia can cause oxygen depletion of the cardiac muscle, and over time result in **myocardial infarction**, or a heart attack.

Blood pressure

Blood pressure is a measure of the pressure the blood exerts against the walls of the blood vessels. Blood pressure readings yield two numbers, the **systolic blood pressure** and the **diastolic blood pressure**. Systolic blood pressure is the maximum pressure exerted by the blood against the arterial walls which occurs at the peak of ventricular contraction. Diastolic blood pressure is the minimum pressure exerted by the blood against the vasculature which occurs at the peak of ventricular relaxation. Blood pressure is usually measured on the upper arm using a **sphygmomanometer (sfig-mo-man-AH-meh-ter)**. The resulting measurement is called the **brachial arterial pressure**. However, blood pressure can be measured at other locations in the body. The ankle is another location where blood pressure is commonly measured. Blood pressure decreases with distance as the blood moves away from the heart. Physicians diagnose peripheral vascular disease (PVD) by examining the ratio of the brachial arterial pressure to the pressure at the ankle.

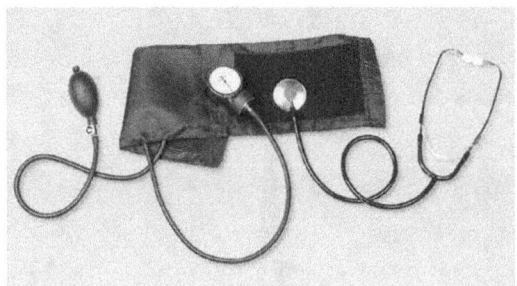

Sphygmomanometer used to measure brachial blood pressure.

Blood pressure is a reflection of the elasticity of the arteries. As arterial resistance increases, so too does the blood pressure. **Arteriosclerosis**, or hardening of the arteries, raises blood pressure and increases the risk of stroke, heart attack, and **aneurism** (bulging of an artery that may ultimately rupture causing death). Blood pressure can change rapidly due to many stimuli: stress, strenuous exercise, smoking, eating, and even a full bladder.

Perfusion Test

Blood must perfuse all of the tissues of the body. Because blood pressure declines with distance away from the heart, perfusion of the extremities is occasionally poor. Without proper blood flow and oxygenation, the fingers and toes lose feeling. Poor perfusion of the tissues can also be an indicator of peripheral vascular disease (PVD). A simple test, called the nail blanch test, is used by physicians to monitor perfusion. The doctor applies pressure to a fingernail until the tissue **blanches**, or turns white. The doctor measures how long it takes for the color to return to the nail bed. A refill time of over two minutes may indicate PVD.

Summary

The cardiovascular system must effectively pump blood into the arterial system, the arteries must maintain enough pressure on the blood to push it through the vascular system and into the tissues, and the blood must enter the capillaries to perfuse the tissue. Medical professionals monitor the body's ability to accomplish these tasks using the pulse, blood pressure, and perfusion tests. The pulse can be measured by palpation or EKG. Blood pressure is measured using a sphygmomanometer. Perfusion is measured using the nail blanch test. The measurements tell the physician how well the heart is functioning, the elasticity of the arteries, and the ability of blood to enter the extremities.

Concept Reinforcement

1. What does an EKG tell a physician and why is it helpful?

2. What is the difference between the systolic and diastolic blood pressure?

3. Describe the nail blanch test. What does an excessively long nail bed refill time tell a physician?

Section 2.3 – The Respiratory System

Section Objective

- Describe the respiratory system and list its key functions

The Respiratory System

The respiratory system consists of the lungs and the airways connecting the lungs to the atmosphere. The airways include the bronchi, the trachea, larynx, pharynx, and nasal passages.

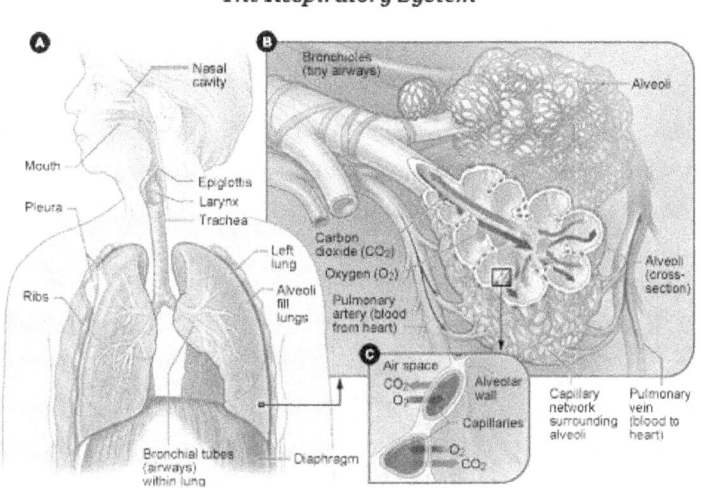

The Respiratory System

The Airways

Air enters the body through the nose and mouth. As air passes through the **nasal passages**, it is warmed and moistened. The **pharynx** connects the **oral cavity** (the inside of the mouth) and nasal passages to the lungs via the **larynx**. It also connects the oral cavity with the **esophagus** (the tube connecting the mouth to the stomach). Air enters the larynx, commonly called the **voice box**, which protects the **trachea** from foreign objects and houses the vocal folds. The trachea conducts warmed, moistened air into the chest where it divides into the two **primary bronchi** (singular, **bronchus**). The bronchi transport air into each lung.

The Lungs

The primary function of the lungs is to serve as the point of gas exchange; carbon dioxide (CO_2) is excreted and oxygen (O_2) is absorbed within the lungs. The lungs may also excrete some of the body's waste products, particularly **ketones**. Ketones are **volatile compounds**, compounds capable of evaporating at room temperature, produced during metabolism of

> A **pro-hormone** is an inactive form of a hormone that becomes a functional hormone after it is metabolized or converted into an active form by special enzymes.

fatty acids when there is insufficient glucose available. **Angiotensin I**, a **pro-hormone**, is converted into **angiotensin II** in the lungs. Angiotensin II causes the blood vessels to constrict, raising blood pressure.

The lungs are served by the two primary bronchi. As the primary bronchi enter the lungs, they branch into **bronchioles**, smaller airways that continue to branch until they terminate in the **alveoli**. The alveoli are small sacs lined with epithelial cells where gas exchange actually occurs. The alveoli increase the surface area over which gasses can be exchanged. In fact, the average person has a surface area nearly as large as a football field folded up into the lungs. The alveolar cells secrete a chemical called **surfactant**, which breaks the surface tension of water allowing the alveoli to inflate. Otherwise, the moisture in the lungs would cause the alveolar walls to stick together. The air in the alveoli must reach 100% humidity so the gasses can dissolve across the cell membranes and enter the blood. Capillaries surround each alveolus, bringing blood as close as it can get to the air for gas exchange.

Summary

The respiratory system consists of the lungs, the bronchi, the trachea, larynx, pharynx, and nasal passages. The air is warmed and moistened to 100% humidity as it passes through the airways into the lungs. The alveoli of the lungs are where gas exchange occurs. The alveoli maximize the surface area over which gas can be exchanged. Capillaries surround each alveolus, bringing blood as close as it can get to the air for gas exchange.

Concept Reinforcement

1. List and describe the major parts of the respiratory system.
2. Describe the importance of the alveoli in the lungs.
3. How are the lungs involved in blood pressure regulation?

Section 2.4 – Lung Volume

Section Objective

- Identify and define several measurements of lung volume

Pulmonary Function

The critical elements in lung function are the ability of the lungs to move air in and out of the lungs and the ability to exchange gasses. To measure these functions, medical professionals measure the total volume of the lungs and how quickly the lungs can move air in and out. The results of these measurements inform physicians of the total lung capacity, the flexibility or stiffness of the lungs, and the possibility of obstructions of the airways. The most important piece of equipment used by physicians to measure lung function is the **spirometer**. A spirometer measures changes in the volume of air. Electronic spirometers are capable of measuring air flow rates in addition to volume changes. Measurements of pulmonary function are different for different ages, races, and sexes. Males tend to have greater lung capacity than females, even when matched for height and weight. Increasing age tends to reduce elasticity, and thus capacity, of the lungs.

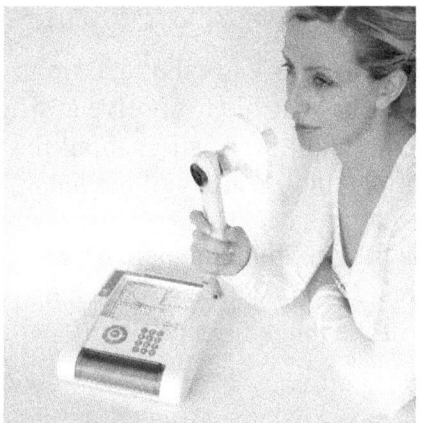

A desktop spirometer

Image courtesy of COSMED

Measurements of Lung Function

Forced vital capacity (FVC) is the maximum amount of air, measured in liters (l), which can be forcibly exhaled after a patient has inhaled the largest breath she is capable of inhaling. FVC helps physicians diagnose obstructive diseases or airway restrictions.

Forced expiratory volume in one second (FEV1) is the volume of air in liters which the patient can forcibly exhale in one second. FEV1 is useful in diagnosing obstructive diseases or airway restrictions.

Forced expiratory volume in three seconds (FEV3) is the volume of air in liters which the patient can forcibly exhale in three seconds. In a healthy patient this should be nearly the entire FVC.

The **FEV1/FVC ratio** combines both the FVC and the FEV1 to give the physician a picture of the ability of the lungs to move air. If the ratio is large, the lungs are capable of moving air easily. If the ratio is small, the lungs are having difficulty moving air, indicating an obstruction or constricted airways.

Similar to the FEV1/FVC ratio, the **FEV3/FVC ratio** combines both the FVC and the FEV3 to give the physician a picture of the ability of the lungs to move air. If the ratio is large, the lungs are capable of moving air easily. If the ratio is small, the lungs are having difficulty moving air, indicating an obstruction or constricted airways.

Peak expiratory flow rate (PEFR) measures the maximum flow rate in liters per second (l/s) at which air is exhaled during a FVC test. This test helps physicians determine whether airways are constricted and whether treatments to dilate the airways, such as asthma treatments, are working.

Forced expiratory flow (FEF) measures the rate at which air is exhaled from the lungs during a FVC test. The FEF is divided into quarters and reported as the FEF25%, FEF50%, and FEF75% because the rate at which air can be expelled from the lungs changes during exhalation.

Maximum voluntary ventilation (MVV) is the total volume of air moved by a patient inhaling and exhaling as rapidly as possible for twelve to fifteen seconds, measured in l/s. This test provides the physician with information about the strength and function of the muscles responsible for breathing, the elasticity of the lungs, and airway resistance.

Total lung capacity (TLC) is the maximum amount of air a patient is capable of inhaling. TLC is commonly used to create ratios with the other lung capacity measurements to determine the relative capacity of the lungs for air.

Summary

Medical professionals measure the total volume of the lungs and how quickly the lungs can move air in and out, the total lung capacity, the flexibility or stiffness of the lungs, and the possibility of obstructions of the airways. Physicians use a spirometer to measure the volume of air moved in liters or liters per second. Forced vital capacity, forced expiratory volume in one second, forced expiratory volume in three seconds, the FEV1/FVC ratio, the FEV3/FVC ratio, peak expiratory flow rate, forced expiratory flow, maximum voluntary ventilation, and total lung capacity are among the most common measurements used by physicians to test lung capacity.

Concept Reinforcement

1. Explain how the **FEV3/FVC ratio** combines both the FVC and the FEV3 to give the physician a picture of the ability of the lungs to move air.

2. What information does a physician derive from the MVV test?

3. How do age and sex affect lung capacity?

Section 2.5 – The Skeletal System

Section Objective

- Define the skeletal system and differentiate between the axial and appendicular skeletal elements

The Skeletal System

The **skeletal system** is made up of the bones, cartilage, ligaments, and tendons that together serve to provide the body with shape, protect the internal organs, and allow the muscles to move the body by providing anchor points against which the muscles can apply leverage. The rigid bones are connected at **joints** where the skeleton allows the body to bend or flex. The joints contain **cartilage**, which serves to cushion the joints, and **ligaments**, which bind the bones together loosely. The muscles are anchored to the bones by strong, elastic connective tissue called **tendons**. The skeletal system composes approximately 20% of the body's total weight.

Bones

The bones provide the body with its overall shape. Without bones, people would be puddles of twitching muscle and organs. The bones also provide the body with support. All of the soft elements of the body are attached to the bones to keep them in their proper place. The bones also serve as a reservoir for **calcium** (Ca), an important mineral used in cell signaling, especially in neurons and muscle cells. The bones are the home for the **hematopoietic stem cells**, the cells that generate the blood supply and immune system. Many people think of the bones as relatively inert and unchanging, basically large rock-like columns upon which the other tissues of the body are hung. However, this is far from true. The bones are constantly adding or extracting Ca to help the body maintain its fine balance of blood Ca levels. Excess or insufficient Ca in the blood can cause **convulsions**, uncontrolled spasmodic muscular contractions, or **tetany**, uncontrolled muscle rigidity. The bones constantly reshape themselves to respond to the stress of activity. For example, people who strength train using weights tend to have larger, stronger bones. This is especially important for women in helping them to avoid osteoporosis later in life. The bones rearrange themselves to orient the crystalline structure of the bone to support the new stress of weight-bearing.

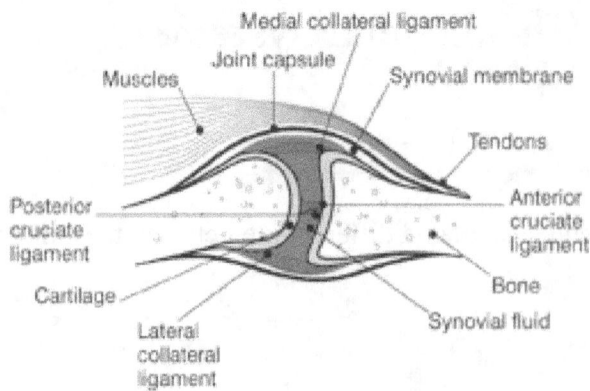

Cartilage serves as a cushion between the bones at a joint. Notice the complexity of even a simple joint such as this one.

Cartilage

Cartilage serves as a cushion between the bones at the joints (see Figure 2 above). Cartilage can serve to provide the body shape, for example the nose and ears. Cartilage creates a template for new bone growth as children grow. The **epiphyseal plates**, segments of cartilage located in the long bones of the arms and legs, create a matrix of cartilage that is invaded by **osteoblasts**, immature bone cells, that will convert the collagen matrix into bone as the bone grows. The matrix is a form or shape of interwoven proteins that serve as a scaffold and mold for the osteoblasts to use to create new bone.

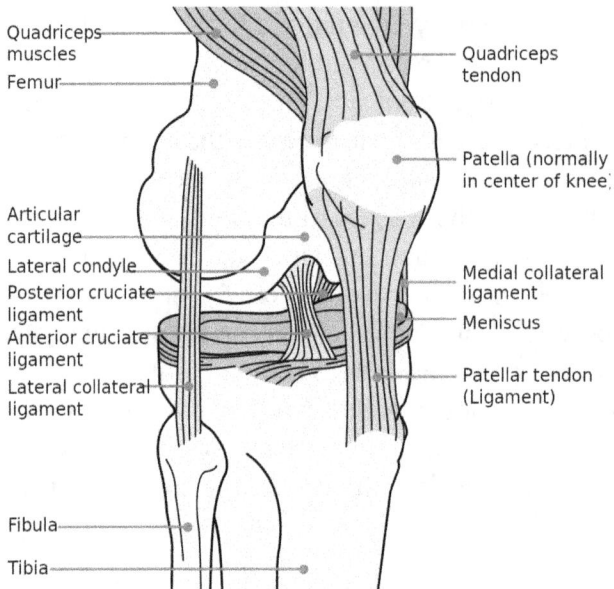

Ligaments

The **ligaments** serve to tie the bones together at the joints and stabilize the joint so that it only moves in the desired direction. Ligaments are made up of dense, inelastic connective tissue. Athletes participate in stretching exercises to make the ligaments of their joints more flexible. Sprains are injuries of the ligaments in which the ligament is stretched too far and may be partially torn. Complete tears are common injuries in many sports, especially tears of the ligaments of the knee. Dislocated joints cause extreme stretching of the ligaments. If not corrected rapidly, it is possible for the ligament to become lax, making the likelihood of future dislocations much greater.

Tendons

Tendons are made up of dense, fibrous connective tissue connecting the muscles to the bones. **Tenocytes**, cells that secrete collagen fibers and collagen fiber binding proteins, create the tendons and can be found packed inside the tendon. Tendons transmit the muscular contractile force to the bones, allowing the muscles to apply force to the bones and generate movement. Tendons must be relatively inelastic to transmit the force as completely as possible. However, tendons are also capable of stretching during movement, storing energy in the same manner as a stiff spring, then releasing the energy. For example, as a runner takes a stride, his leg strikes the ground and flexes. As part of the flexing, tendons stretch, storing energy. As the runner pushes off in the next stride, the energy stored in the tendons is released, reducing the amount of muscular energy required to run.

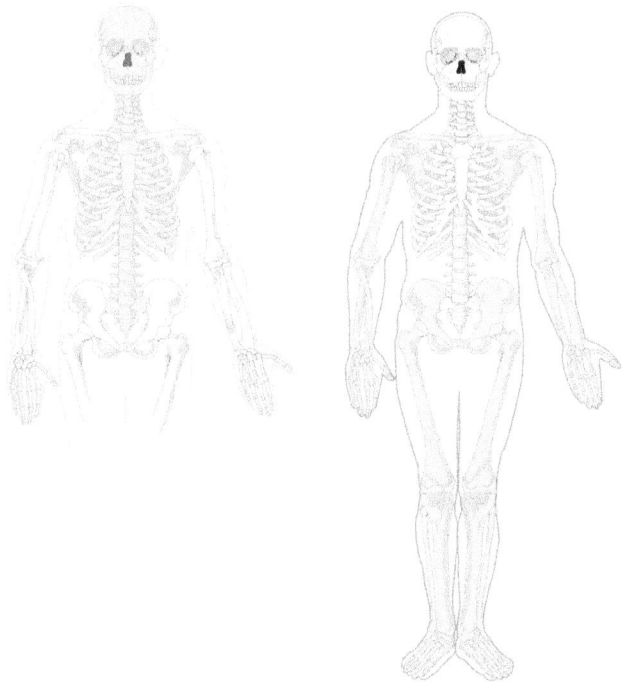

The axial (left) and appendicular (right) skeletal elements can be seen above. The appendicular elements include the extremities and the bones connecting them to the axial elements. The axial elements include the bones responsible for protecting the vital organs and providing the axis of the body.

Axial and Appendicular Skeletal Elements

The skeleton consists of 206 bones divided into the 80 bones of the axial skeletal elements and the 126 bones of the appendicular skeletal elements. The **axial elements** include the bones of the skull, vertebral column, ribs, and sternum. The **appendicular elements** include the bones of the **extremities**, arms, legs, hands, and feet, and the bones that connect the extremities to the axial skeletal elements, called **girdles**. The **pelvic girdle** connects the legs to the vertebral column via the bones of the hip and the **pectoral girdle** attaches the arms to the ribs, vertebral column and sternum via the **clavicles**, or collar bones, and the **scapulae** (singular: **scapula**), or the shoulder blades.

Summary

The skeletal system is made up of the bones, cartilage, ligaments, and tendons that together serve to provide the body with shape, protect the internal organs, and allow the muscles to move the body at the joints by providing anchor points against which the muscles can apply leverage. The bones provide the body with shape and support, serve as a reservoir for Ca, and are home for the hematopoietic stem cells. Cartilage serves as a cushion between the bones at the joints, provides the body shape, and creates a template for new bone growth as children grow. The ligaments serve to tie the bones together at the joints and stabilize the joint so that it only moves in the desired direction. Tendons transmit the contractile force of the muscles to the bones, allowing the muscles to apply force to the bones and generate movement. The skeleton consists of axial skeletal elements, which include the bones of the skull, vertebral column, ribs, and sternum, and the appendicular skeletal elements, which include the bones of the extremities and their girdles.

Concept Reinforcement

1. List three functions of bone.

2. Explain the difference between ligaments and tendons.

3. List the primary components of the axial and appendicular skeletal systems.

Section 2.6 – Bone Tissue and Bone Health

Section Objectives

- Describe the types and features of bone tissue and the functions of each
- Discuss bone density and how it can affect athletic performance and general health

Types of Bone Tissue

Bone is made up of two different types of **osseous**, or bony, tissue: **cortical bone**, or compact bone, and **cancellous bone**, or spongy bone, also called **trabecular bone**. Both cortical bone and cancellous bone provide structure and support to the body, provide levers upon which the muscles can act to move the body, protect the vital organs, and serve as a storage depot for minerals.

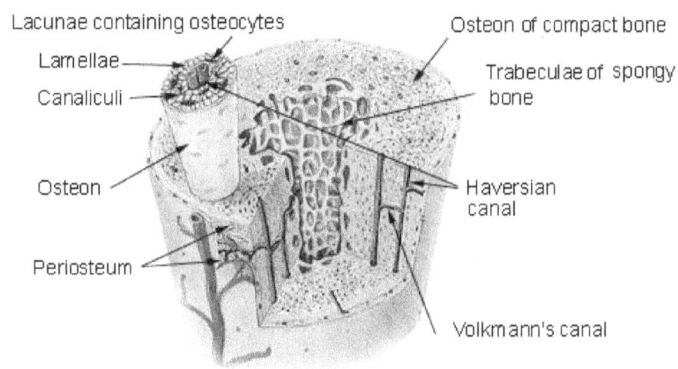

Cortical Bone

Cortical bone makes up the outer perimeter of a bone. Cortical bone is composed of densely packed columns of **osteons**. Osteons are composed of **osteocytes**, mature bone cells, **collagen fibers**, protein fibers that serves as a scaffold and which are found in most connective tissue, and **hydroxyapatite crystals**, calcium phosphate crystals that are the primary form of calcium deposits in the bone. Cortical bone serves as the hard outer layer of a bone, protecting the less dense interior of the bone. The long bones of the arms and legs contain long hollow shafts enclosed in layers of cortical bone. The hollow region contains bone marrow. The dense cortical bone ensures that bone marrow remains sequestered, or stored and kept separate from the rest of the body, in the bone.

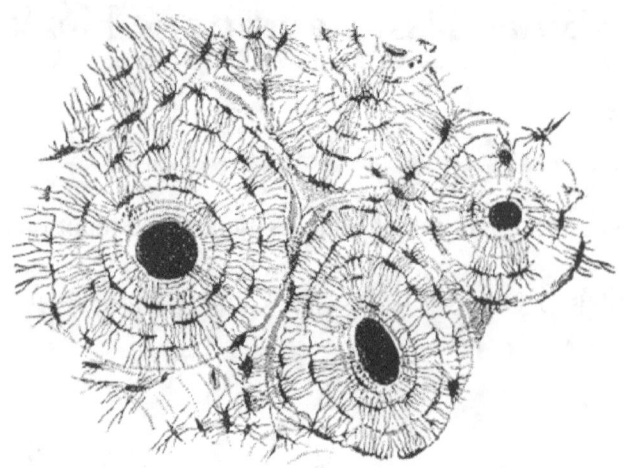

The photomicrograph of bone above shows bone structure. Notice the regular circular shape of the osteons. Each osteon is composed of osteocytes, collagen fibers, and hydroxyapatite crystals.

Cancellous Bone

Cancellous bone, also called trabecular bone, is spongy in appearance only, not texture. Cancellous bone fills the less dense interior of the bones. Cancellous bone is called trabecular bone because of its numerous **trabeculae** (singular trabecula), tiny strut-like bridges that create numerous hollow spaces within the bone. Cancellous bone is home to the red bone marrow where **hematopoietic stem cells**, the cells that give rise to all of the cells of the blood, reside. Cancellous bone is where the majority of the arteries and veins within the bone are found.

The Importance of Bone Density

Athletes rely on strong bones to perform at a high level. The stresses athletes place on their bones can cause them to fracture even in the absence of a blow if the bones are not dense and strong. In the case of athletes with low bone densities, even the impact of landing after a jump can result in a bone fracture. **Bone density** is a measure of the level of **calcification**, or calcium deposition, of the bones. Bone density is one way to determine the strength of bones. The greater the calcification of the bone, the stronger it usually is. Bones that have low density, are more prone to **fracture**, or breaking, than dense bones.

Bone density decreases as we age in a process called **osteopenia**. The calcium is mobilized from the bone faster than it is deposited as we grow older. The problem is especially important in postmenopausal women, who suffer disproportionately from **osteoporosis**. Osteoporosis is a reduction in bone density as a result of calcium loss in the bone. However, men also suffer from the disease. Resistance training with weights combined with calcium supplementation is a good way to increase bone density in both women and men. Women who enter menopause with denser bones are less likely to suffer from osteoporosis.

Many female athletes suffer from osteoporosis because of a combination of excessive exercise and inadequate nutrition. Adolescent female athletes in particular are likely to consume too few calories and insufficient calcium for optimum bone growth and density. There are numerous reports of female athletes and dancers who have bone densities similar to women in their 80's. Female athletes and their coaches and trainers should be especially careful to maintain optimum bone density to avoid osteoporosis and its resultant injuries.

Normal Bone 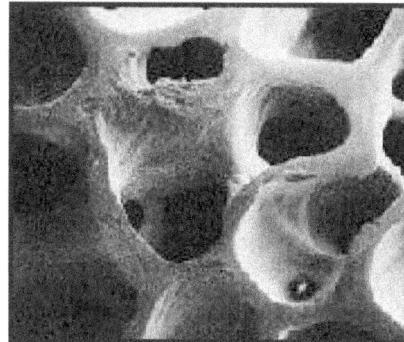 Osteoporotic Bone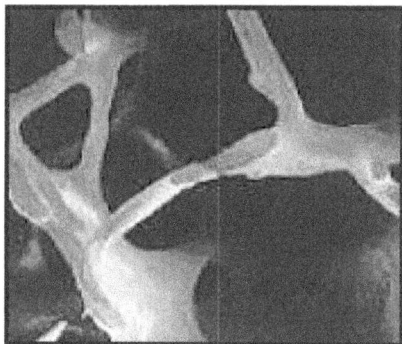

Reproduced from J Bone Miner Res 1986;1:16-21 with permission of the American Society for Bone and Mineral Research.

Summary

Bone is made up of two different types of osseous tissue: cortical bone and cancellous bone. Both types of osseous tissue provide structure and support to the body, provide levers upon which the muscles can act to move the body, protect the vital organs, and serve as a storage depot for minerals. Cortical bone is composed of densely packed columns of osteons. Osteons are composed of osteocytes, collagen fibers, and hydroxyapatite crystals. Cortical bone serves as the hard outer layer of a bone, protecting the less dense interior of the bone. The long bones of the arms and legs contain long, hollow, marrow-filled shafts enclosed in dense cortical bone which ensures that bone marrow remains sequestered in the bone. Cancellous bone fills the less dense interior of the bones with tiny strut-like bridges called trabeculae. Cancellous bone is home to the red bone marrow where hematopoietic stem cells reside, and the majority of the arteries and veins within the bone.

Athletes rely on strong bones to perform at a high level. The stresses athletes place on their bones can cause them to fracture even in the absence of a blow if the bones are not dense and strong. Osteoporosis is a reduction in bone density as a result of calcium loss in the bone. Many female athletes suffer from osteoporosis because of a combination of excessive exercise and inadequate nutrition. Female athletes and their coaches and trainers should be especially careful to maintain optimum bone density to avoid osteoporosis and its resultant injuries.

Concept Reinforcement

1. What are the differences between cortical bone and cancellous bone?

2. List the functions cortical bone and cancellous bone share.

3. Describe osteoporosis and explain why athletes should be concerned about bone density.

Section 2.7 – The Stress-Strain Curve

Section Objective

- Discuss the Stress-Strain curve and list its four phases

The Stress-Strain Curve

The **Stress-Strain curve** is a graphical representation of the strength of an object when it is placed under a load and how the object deforms as a result of that load. Stress-Strain curves are commonly seen in mechanical engineering applications where the ability of an item such as a beam to carry a specified load without bending, stretching, compressing, or failing is critical to safety and its function. There are four major phases in the Stress-Strain curve: yield strength, strain hardening, necking, and rupture. For brittle objects such as glass, any deformation results in rupture, so yield strength and rupture are the same. There is no strain hardening or necking.

In sports medicine, the Stress-Strain curve is used to measure the ability of bones, ligaments, and tendons to bear the loads placed upon them by athletic competition. Tendons and ligaments are capable of stretching to some degree, but do not undergo compression. Bones, although typically thought of as brittle, have the capacity to flex slightly and are compressible.

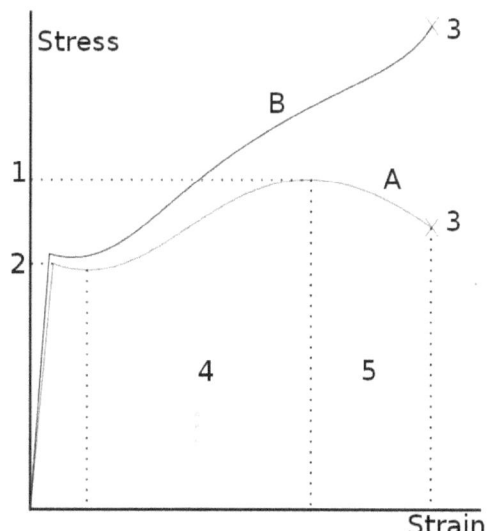

A Stress-Strain curve showing the ultimate strength (1), the yield strength (2), rupture point (3), strain hardening region (4), and necking region (5) for a sample under stress. The blue line represents the "true stress" versus "true strain". The red line represents an engineering Stress-Strain curve: the change in the stress on the sample as it deforms to take the load. Deformation of a sample can actually reduce the stress on the sample even though the strain on the sample increases.

Yield Strength

The **yield strength** of a sample is the strain the sample can support without **deforming plastically**. **Deformation** is any change in the structure of the sample including compression, bending, or stretching. **Elastic deformation** is the level of deformation to which a sample can be subjected and still return to its original shape. **Plastic deformation** is deformation that occurs beyond this point; the sample cannot return to its original shape.

Strain-Hardening Region

The **strain hardening region** of the Stress-Strain curve is the region in which the sample actually becomes stronger as a result of the forces placed upon it. When bone is compressed, for example, it actually becomes harder because the force applied to the bone is dispersed over the entire volume of the bone and each element of the bone presses against the others. The individual components all become stiffer, but because none have failed at this point, each presses equally strongly against the others, and the bone's strength increases. Strain-hardening increases until the **ultimate strength** of the sample is reached. The ultimate strength of a sample is the maximum stress it can bear when subjected to tension, compression, or shearing.

Necking Region

The **necking region** of the Stress-Strain curve is the region in which one segment of the sample abruptly loses diameter and forms a "neck." The sample becomes narrower with a concomitant loss of strength. On the "true" Stress-Strain curve, the stress increases, on the engineering Stress-Strain curve the stress decreases because stress across the whole sample declines even though it increases significantly at the neck.

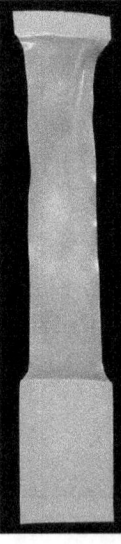

This polyethylene material has been stretched to form a neck. The polyethylene will never regain its former shape.

Rupture

Rupture occurs when the neck becomes unstable and can no longer support the load. In the case of samples that rupture after plastic deformation, the sample pieces cannot be put back together in the same way in which they were originally configured. For brittle samples, the object can be put back together as it was before rupture. Bones, for example, are essentially brittle in this context and can be put back together in much the same way they were before breaking. Ligaments and tendons, on the other hand, undergo plastic deformation and will not return to exactly the same shape and size after healing.

Stresses in Athletics

Stresses and strain are placed on tendons, ligaments, and bones during athletic competition. Athletes are often required to lift heavy objects, such as in Olympic weight lifting, exert high torque on ligaments and tendons, such as when throwing or kicking a ball, and absorb impacts, as seen in football, rugby, and ice hockey. Sudden changes in direction, commonly seen in basketball and soccer, can create enormous stress on ligaments and tendons in the ankles and knees. Trainers use their knowledge of the Stress-Strain curve to design appropriate training programs so that athletes' ligaments and tendons have a chance to adapt to the stresses being placed upon them gradually. In this way, they are able to bear the load rather than stretch or tear. Sports equipment manufacturers calculate the forces being generated against bones and other body structures to design protective gear that dissipates the force of the blow sufficiently to prevent broken bones.

Summary

The Stress-Strain curve is a graphical representation of the strength of an object when it is placed under a load and how the object deforms as a result of that load. There are four major phases in the Stress-Strain curve: yield strength, strain hardening, necking, and rupture. For brittle objects such as glass, any deformation results in rupture, so yield strength and rupture are the same. In sports medicine, the Stress-Strain curve is used to measure the ability of bones, ligaments, and tendons to bear the loads placed upon them by athletic competition. The yield strength of a sample is the strain the sample can support without deforming plastically. The strain hardening region of the Stress-Strain curve is the region in which the sample actually becomes stronger as a result of the forces placed upon it. The necking region of the Stress-Strain curve is the region in which one segment of the sample abruptly loses diameter and forms a "neck". Rupture occurs when the neck becomes unstable and can no longer support the load. Bones are essentially brittle and can be put back together in much the same way they were before breaking. Ligaments and tendons, on the other hand, undergo plastic deformation and will not return to exactly the same shape and size after healing.

Concept Reinforcement

1. Explain why the Stress-Strain curve is useful in sports medicine.

2. Describe the difference between Yield Strength and Ultimate Strength.

3. Contrast rupture of a brittle sample to rupture of a non-brittle sample.

Section 2.8 – Joints and Levers

Section Objective

- Describe a typical joint and discuss the three classes of levers

The Typical Skeletal Joint

Joints are the flexible points between bones that permit the body to move. If there were no joints between the bones, the body would be a single rigid structure similar to a building. A typical joint is composed of several different tissues including bone, cartilage, ligaments, tendons, and joint capsules, and are filled with synovial fluid. Non-typical joints would include the joints between the bones of the skull, which do not permit movement, but rather **suture**, or tie, bones together.

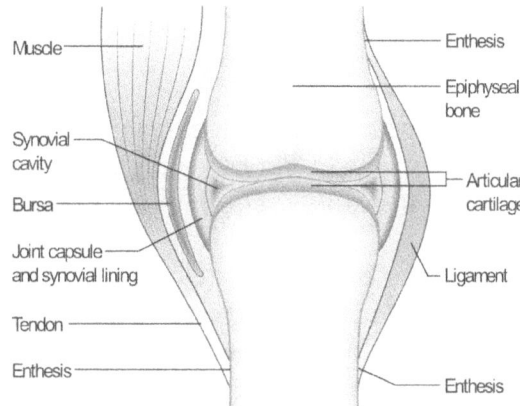

A typical joint in the skeleton contains bone, cartilage, ligaments, tendons, and a joint capsule. The space between the bones is filled with synovial fluid to lubricate the joint.

The Anatomy of a Joint

The bone at a typical joint in the skeleton consists primarily of **cancellous bone**, or spongy bone. The bone forms a head-shaped terminus, called the **epiphysis**, which can insert into a socket or roll across a similarly shaped epiphysis on the end of the next bone. The epiphysis is overlain by a layer of **articular cartilage**, or cartilage of a joint. The articular cartilage serves to reduce the friction at the joint and absorb some of the impact between bones that can occur at a joint, for example, during walking. The entire joint is surrounded by the tough, fibrous **joint capsule**. The **joint capsule** is composed of an outer fibrous connective tissue layer and the inner synovial membrane. The **synovial membrane** secretes **synovial fluid**, a watery fluid that serves as a lubricant between the joints. Synovial fluid also maintains the cartilage in a hydrated state. **Ligaments** made up of tough, relatively inelastic connective tissue, serve to bind the bones to each other and stabilize the movement of the joint. **Tendons**, also made up of tough, relatively inelastic connective tissue, anchor the muscles to the bones and apply muscular force to the bones to create movement at the joints.

Levers

There are three basic classes of levers found at the joints of the skeleton. **First class levers** possess a **fulcrum**, a pivot point around which a lever moves, which is located between the force and the load. An example of a first class lever in the body would be the elbow joint of the arm extending because of the triceps muscle. This type of lever moves relatively slowly, but applies greater force to the load.

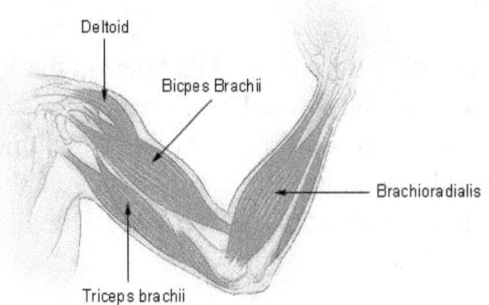

The triceps brachii is an example of a first class lever in the body.
The biceps brachii is an example of a third class lever.

Second class levers the load is between the fulcrum and the point at which the force is applied. This type of lever moves slowly, but can apply great force to the load. A second class lever in the body would be the calf muscle, or **gastrocnemius**, flexing the foot.

Third class levers apply the force between the fulcrum and the load. This type of lever cannot apply as much force to the load, but results in rapid movement. Flexing of the elbow by the biceps muscle is an example of a third class lever in the body.

Summary

A typical joint is composed of several different tissues including bone, cartilage, ligaments, tendons, and joint capsules, and are filled with synovial fluid. The epiphysis at the end of the bone inserts into a socket or rolls across a similarly shaped epiphysis on the end of the next bone. The epiphysis is overlain by a layer of articular cartilage which serves to reduce the friction at the joint and absorb some of the impact between bones. The entire joint is surrounded by the joint capsule which is composed of an outer fibrous connective tissue layer and the inner synovial membrane. The synovial membrane secretes synovial fluid to lubricate the joints and maintains the cartilage in a hydrated state. Ligaments serve to bind the bones to each other and stabilize the movement of the joint. Tendons anchor the muscles to the bones and apply muscular force to the bones to create movement at the joints. There are three basic classes of levers found at the joints of the skeleton. In a first-class lever, the fulcrum is located between the force and the load. In a second-class lever, the load is between the fulcrum and the applied force. In a third-class lever, the force is applied between the fulcrum and the load.

Concept Reinforcement

1. List the seven components of a joint.

2. Describe the difference between a first class lever and a second class lever. Provide an example from the body of each.

3. Describe the difference between a first class lever and a third class. Provide an example from the body of each

Section 2.9 – The Muscular System

Section Objective

- Define the muscular system and describe the three types of muscle tissue

The Muscular System

The muscular system is composed of the specialized contractile cells called **myocytes**, or muscle cells, which make movement of the body and within the body possible. A **contractile cell** is one that is capable of **contracting**, or shortening itself. Most people readily think of external movements such as walking or throwing as functions of the muscular system, but breathing, movement of food, and circulation of the blood are examples of movements within the body which rely upon muscle contractions. Posture stabilization and facial expressions are other critical functions of the muscular system. The muscular system generates approximately 85% of the heat produced by the body.

The muscular system is under the control of the nervous system. Portions of the muscular system are under voluntary control while other portions are controlled by the **autonomic**, or involuntary, nervous system. Neurons, or nerve cells, release chemicals at **neuromuscular junctions** which cause myocytes to contract. Because myocytes contract in order to cause movement, muscles _**always pull, they never push.**_

Muscle Tissue

There are three types of muscle tissue in the body: **smooth muscle**, **striated muscle**, and **cardiac muscle**. Each type differs significantly from the other and each is specialized to carry out very different tasks optimally. All muscle tissue contains two proteins which are responsible for contraction: **actin** and **myosin**. Muscle contracts when the two molecules slide past one another, the **sliding filament model** of muscle contraction. The myosin binds to actin filaments, then flexes to slide the actin and myosin filaments past one another. The myosin then releases the actin filament and reattaches further down the actin filament to repeat the process.

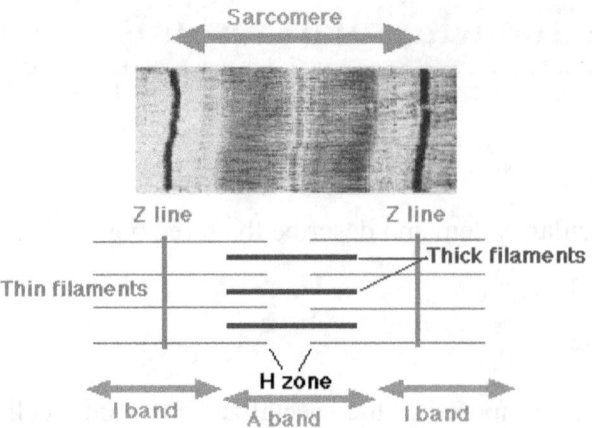

The photomicrograph of a sarcomere above is reproduced as a labeled line drawing. A sarcomere is the unit of the muscle cell from one Z line to the next Z line. The bands of the sarcomere exist because of the overlapping arrangement of the muscle proteins. The Z line serves as the anchor point for the actin filaments. The thick filaments of the A band are the myosin filaments. When the muscle contracts, the sarcomere length is reduced, the Z bands move toward one another, and the H zone and I bands disappear.

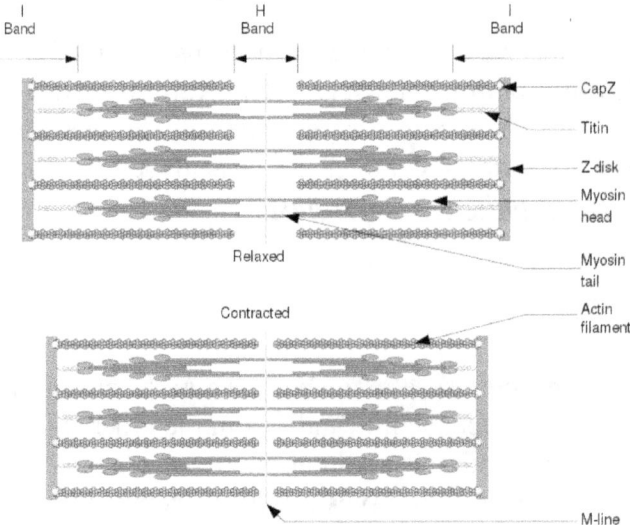

The sliding filament model of muscle contraction states that muscles contract because the actin and myosin filaments slide past one another to shorten the cell.

Smooth Muscle

Smooth muscle is the muscle responsible for involuntary activities such as movement of food through the digestive tract, blood pressure regulation, and some reproductive functions. Smooth muscle is stimulated by the **autonomic nervous system**, the portion of the nervous system that is not under voluntary control. Smooth muscle cells are spindle-shaped. The nucleus of smooth muscle cells is usually located in the center of the cell. The actin and myosin chains are not arranged in any specific pattern within the cell, but rather as loosely arranged sheets. They are attached to the cell membrane and the cell **cytoskeleton**, the protein fibers within a cell that give it its characteristic shape and provide support.

In addition to autonomic neural control of contraction, smooth muscle has the interesting property of contracting when something stretches the tissue. For example, as food enters the intestine, the intestine stretches to accommodate the food. The smooth muscle of the intestine contracts to push the food along the digestive tract. Both the autonomic nervous system and the stretch-induced contraction of the intestinal smooth muscle are responsible for moving food along the digestive tract.

Striated Muscle

Striated muscle is also known as **skeletal muscle**, or **voluntary muscle**. Striated muscle is under voluntary control by the central nervous system. Striated muscle is so called because the arrangement of the filaments is such that distinct banding patterns can be detected easily with the aid of a microscope. Muscle cells in striated muscle are called **myofibers** or **muscle fibers**. Myofibers are **multinucleate** cells whose multiple nuclei are located just beneath the plasma membrane. Myofibers contain many more **mitochondria**, the powerhouses of cells, than an average cell possesses. Myofibers are packed densely with **myofibrils**, the proteins arranged as a long series of individual **sarcomeres**.

The actin and myosin filaments within the myofibers are arranged in **sarcomeres**, the special functional unit of striated muscle. The sarcomere consists of two Z lines, two I bands, an A band, and an H zone. The **Z line** serves as the anchor point for the actin filaments. A single sarcomere is the group of proteins from one Z line to the next Z line. The **I bands** are the region of the sarcomere containing actin filaments. The **A band** is the region of the sarcomere containing overlapping actin and myosin filaments. The **H zone** is the region of the sarcomere which contains only the tails of the myosin filaments. The tails of the myosin filaments on the left side are bound to the tails of the myosin filaments on the right side. When the muscle contracts the sarcomeres shorten as the filaments slide past one another. The H zone and I bands disappear while the Z lines move toward one another.

Cardiac Muscle

Cardiac muscle possesses characteristics of both smooth muscle and striated muscle. Like smooth muscle, cardiac muscle is not under voluntary control. Cardiac muscle is innervated by the autonomic nervous system, also similar to smooth muscle. Like striated muscle, cardiac muscle is striated in appearance, with actin and myosin filaments aligned as in striated muscle, but with **T lines** instead of Z lines which anchor the actin filaments in place. Similar to striated muscle, cardiomyocytes, cardiac muscle cells, contain many mitochondria. Unlike the multinucleate, cylindrically shaped, striated myofibers, cardiomyocytes are **mononucleate**, possessing only one nucleus, and they may be branched. Cardiac muscle contains **intercalated discs** which serve to identify cardiac muscle when viewed under a microscope. Intercalated discs are specialized structures which join cardiomyocytes together and help **propagate**, or spread, action potentials, or nerve signals. Intercalated discs help ensure the heart beats in a synchronized fashion to pump blood. Cardiomyocytes have the unique property of self stimulation. They will contract in the absence of a neural signal to do so. However, the heart cannot beat in a synchronized fashion without neural signals. Instead, it will quiver, a condition called **fibrillation**.

Summary

The muscular system is composed of myocytes, which make movement of the body and within the body possible. Movements include walking, throwing, breathing, movement of food, circulation of the blood, posture stabilization, and facial expressions. The muscular system generates approximately 85% of the heat produced by the body. Portions of the muscular system are under voluntary control while other portions are controlled by the autonomic, or involuntary, nervous system. Muscles <u>always pull, they never push.</u> There are three types of muscle tissue in the body: smooth muscle, striated muscle, and cardiac muscle. All muscle tissue contains actin and myosin. Muscle contracts when the two molecules slide past one another. Smooth muscle is the muscle responsible for involuntary activities. Smooth muscle is stimulated by the autonomic nervous system and being stretched. Smooth muscle cells are spindle-shaped, with a centrally located nucleus and irregularly arranged actin and myosin filaments. Striated muscle is under voluntary control. Myofibers are multinucleate cells which contain many mitochondria and are packed densely with myofibrils. The actin and myosin filaments within the myofibers are arranged in sarcomeres, the special functional unit of striated muscle. When the muscle contracts the sarcomeres shorten as the filaments slide past one another. Cardiac muscle possesses characteristics of both smooth muscle and striated muscle. Like smooth muscle, cardiac muscle is not under voluntary control, mononucleate, and innervated by the autonomic nervous system. Cardiac muscle is striated in appearance and contains many mitochondria. Cardiomyocytes may be branched and contain intercalated discs. Intercalated discs help propagate action potentials to ensure the heart beats in a synchronized fashion to pump blood. Cardiomyocytes have the unique property of self stimulation, but the heart will fibrillate without external neural signals.

Concept Reinforcement

1. Describe the general structure of the muscular system.

2. List the differences between smooth and striated muscle.

3. List the similarities between cardiac and striated muscle.

Section 2.10 – The Central Nervous System

Section Objective

- Describe the central nervous system and describe its role in bodily functions

The Central Nervous System

The **central nervous system** (CNS) is composed of the brain and the spinal cord. The brain and spinal cord are composed of neurons and a number of supporting cells called **glia**, including oligodendrocytes and astrocytes. **Oligodendrocytes** cover the neurons of the CNS with myelin, increasing the speed with which neural signals can be transmitted. **Astrocytes** are star-shaped glial cells which serve as the immune system of the CNS, provide nutrients to the neurons of the CNS, and form an important part of the **blood-brain barrier** (BBB). The BBB is a selective barrier that only permits certain molecules to enter the central nervous system. The CNS is covered by a tough layer of tissue called the **meninges**. The meninges are made up of three distinct layers which carry the blood vessels that nourish the brain and provide a physical cushion for the brain against the bones of the skull. **Meningitis** is an inflammation of the meninges and is frequently fatal.

Role of the CNS

The Brain

The brain is the master controller of the body. All neural signals are ultimately relayed to the brain for processing. Signals from the brain are relayed to the other parts of the body to effect movement and changes in the body's function. The brain directly **innervates**, or supplies neural input to, the body via the twelve **cranial nerves**. The sense of smell is mediated by the **olfactory epithelium** in the nasal passages. The olfactory epithelium provides the brain with information about chemicals through their odors via the **olfactory nerve**, cranial nerve I. Visual stimuli reach the brain via the second cranial nerve (II), the **optic nerve**. The movement of the eyes is controlled by the **oculomotor nerve**, cranial nerve III, the **trochlear nerve**, cranial nerve IV, and the **abducens nerve**, cranial nerve VI. The **trigeminal nerve**, cranial nerve V, receives sensory input from the face and controls the muscles of **mastication**, or chewing. The **facial nerve**, cranial nerve VII, controls facial expressions, the tear glands, and salivary glands, and is involved in relaying taste sensations from the tongue. Sounds and information about balance are transmitted to the brain via the **vestibulochoclear nerve**, cranial nerve VIII. Taste is relayed to the brain by the **glossopharyngeal nerve**, cranial nerve IX, which also controls salivary glands. The **vagus nerve**, cranial nerve X, activates the muscles in the larynx and pharynx beneath the oral cavity and is involved in speech control. It supplies autonomic innervation to thorax and abdomen. Cranial nerve XI, the **accessory nerve**, controls the muscles of the neck. Finally, the **hypoglossal nerve**, cranial nerve XII, controls the tongue and is important in swallowing and speech.

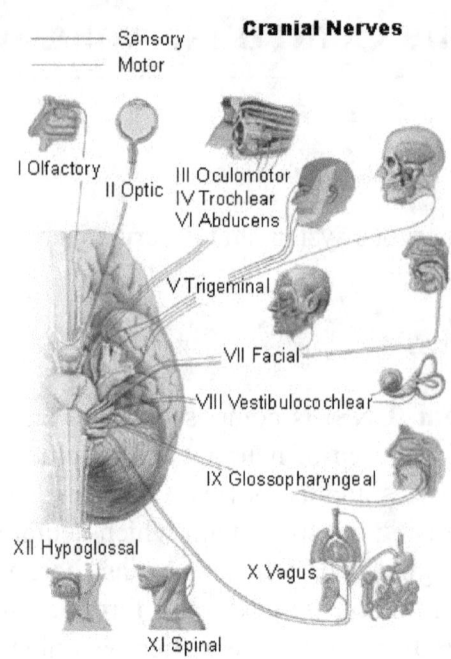

The Spinal Cord

The brain controls the rest of the body via the spinal cord. The neurons of the brain (other than the cranial nerves) extend axons through the base of the skull via the **foramen magnum**, the hole at the junction of the skull and the **atlas**, which is first vertebra of the vertebral column. The axons do not extend the entire length of the vertebral column. Instead, they terminate on neurons in the grey matter which exit the spinal column at the lower lumbar and sacral vertebrae in what is called the **cauda equina**, or horse's tail, because it resembles a horse's tail in appearance.

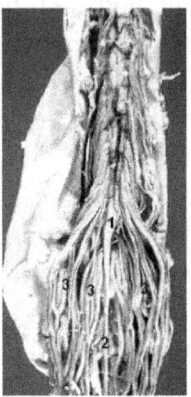

Anterior view of a human cauda equine. 1. Conus medullaris 2. Filum terminale 3. Cauda equine. Note the resemblance of the nerves to a horse's tail. Image courtesy of John A Beal, PhD, Department of Cellular Biology & Anatomy, Louisiana State University Health Sciences Center, Shreveport.

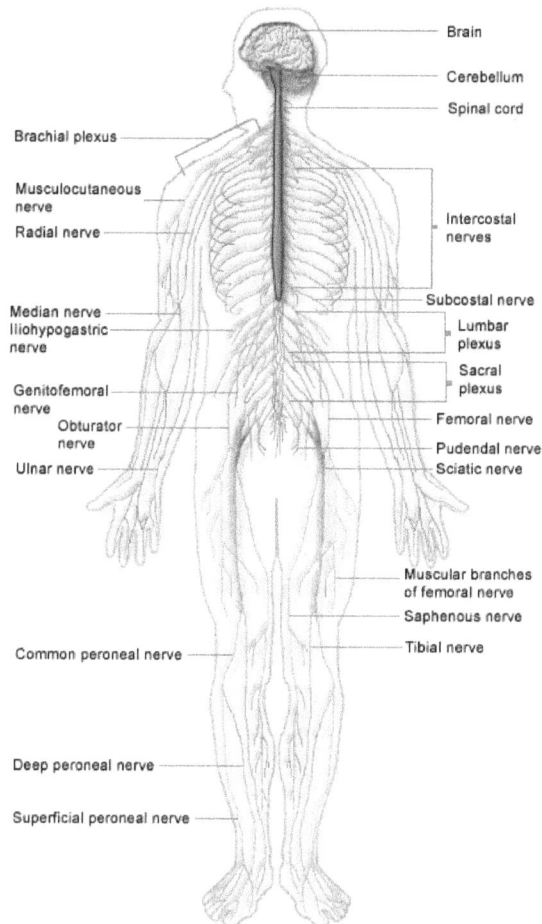

The spinal cord consists of **grey matter** and **white matter**. The axons from the brain terminate on the **efferent motor neurons**, neurons which carry signals for muscular movement from the spinal cord to the body. The efferent motor neurons form the **grey matter** of the spinal cord. The **white matter** of the spinal cord consists of the myelinated axons from the brain or from the **afferent sensory neurons** from the **dorsal root ganglia**. **Afferent sensory neurons** carry sensory signals from the body toward the brain. The dorsal root ganglia are small clusters of sensory neuron cell bodies which project axons into the spinal cord.

The spinal cord is not solely a pipeline of information. **Reflexes** are actions that occur almost instantly, that are often executed by voluntary muscles, and that are not under voluntary control. These actions are controlled within the spinal cord. A **reflex arc** occurs when an afferent sensory neuron stimulates an efferent motor neuron within the spinal cord to generate movement. The stimulus is relayed to the brain, but by the time the brain has registered the stimulus, the body has already moved. The **knee jerk** reflex is the reflex most commonly tested by a doctor when he strikes the knee with a small rubber hammer.

Summary

The CNS is composed of the brain and the spinal cord. The brain and spinal cord are composed of neurons and glia, including oligodendrocytes and astrocytes. Oligodendrocytes cover the neurons of the CNS with myelin, while astrocytes serve as the immune system of the CNS, provide nutrients to the neurons of the CNS, and form an important part of the BBB. The BBB is a selective barrier that only permits certain molecules to enter the central nervous system. The CNS is covered by a tough layer of tissue called the meninges which are made up of three distinct layers carrying the blood vessels that nourish the brain and providing a physical cushion for the brain against the bones of the skull. The brain is the master controller of the body. All neural signals are ultimately relayed to the brain for processing. The brain directly innervates the body via the twelve cranial nerves: the olfactory nerve, optic nerve, oculomotor nerve, trochlear nerve, abducens nerve, trigeminal nerve, facial nerve, vestibulochoclear nerve, glossopharyngeal nerve, vagus nerve, accessory nerve, and the hypoglossal nerve. The brain controls the rest of the body via the spinal cord. The spinal cord consists of grey matter and white matter. The neurons of the brain (other than the cranial nerves) extend axons through the base of the skull via the foramen magnum, to terminate on the efferent motor neurons in the grey matter which carry signals for muscular movement from the spinal cord to the body. The white matter of the spinal cord consists of the myelinated axons from the brain or from the afferent sensory neurons which carry sensory signals from the body toward the brain. The spinal cord terminates on neurons which exit the spinal column at the lower lumbar and sacral vertebrae in the cauda equine. Reflexes are controlled within the spinal cord. A reflex arc occurs when an afferent sensory neuron stimulates an efferent motor neuron within the spinal cord to generate movement.

Concept Reinforcement

1. What are the components of the central nervous system?

2. List the twelve cranial nerves.

3. Explain how a reflex arc works.

Section 2.11 – The FIT Principle

Section Objective

- Describe the FIT principle

The FIT Principle

The FIT principle is a tool used by trainers to help individuals and athletes develop training programs to reach their goals. FIT stands for **frequency**, **intensity**, and **time**. Trainers develop exercise programs based on how often, or frequency, exertion level, or intensity, and number of minutes, or time, a person should exercise. By varying the frequency, intensity, and time of the exercises performed, individuals and athletes can achieve very different goals for their bodies, health, and fitness levels using exercise. Each of the three components of the FIT principle is related to the others and must be considered in conjunction with the others when developing an exercise plan.

Frequency

The frequency with which exercise is performed depends upon the intensity of the exercise performed and the length of time for which it is performed. Experts recommend that everyone should exercise every day for at least 30 minutes to maintain good general health. In general, this recommendation refers to low intensity exercise such as walking, active stretching, or some other light exercise. While this is sufficient for the general population to maintain health, it is not enough to promote weight loss or improve athletic performance.

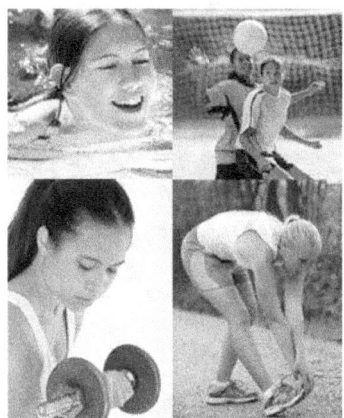

By varying the type of activity and its intensity, exercise frequency can be kept high while avoiding injury or overtraining.

To improve athletic performance, exercise is generally performed at higher intensities or longer duration. In either case, daily exercise may be excessive. Exercise causes damage, microtears, to the muscle cells, tendons, and ligaments of the body. The body repairs the damage and at the same time increases the size of the muscle or improves its aerobic capacity. The body strengthens ligaments, tendons, and bones. The body must have sufficient time to perform these repairs. High intensity or long duration exercise performed too frequently, overtraining, will result in weakening of the muscles, loss of muscle mass, and damage to the ligaments and tendons. Athletes vary their exercise plan each day to avoid overtraining injuries. For example, Monday, Wednesday, and Friday may be strength training days while Tuesday, Thursday, and Saturday may be aerobic training days, and Sunday may be a day of rest.

Intensity

Exercise intensity asks the question, "How hard are you working?" High intensity aerobic exercise increases the heart rate and is usually measured using a heart rate monitor. The maximum heart rate is the fastest rate the heart is capable of beating. It can be estimated by the formula: 220 - age = maximum heart rate. Exercise intensity is then calculated as a percentage of the maximum heart rate. High intensity aerobic workouts generally utilize a heart rate that is 80 to 90% of maximum, moderate intensity workouts use between 70 and 80%, and low intensity workouts use between 60 and 70% as their target heart rates.

Strength training using weights may or may not elevate heart rate significantly, depending upon the method used. Rapid circuit training can elevate heart rate significantly. Power lifting, on the other hand, does little to increase heart rate. The intensity of strength training is generally determined using the amount of weight, the number of sets, and the number of repetitions within each set. Heavier weights, more explosive movement, high repetitions, and more sets increase the intensity of a workout. Generally speaking, as the number of sets and repetitions increases, the weight decreases. Explosive movements are usually performed using the body's weight or intermediate weights.

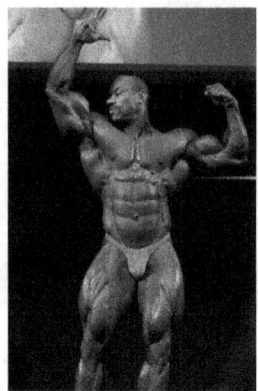

Dexter Jackson, Mr. Olympia 2008.

Photo by: LocalFitness.com.au

Time

The amount of time spent exercising each day depends upon the frequency and intensity of exercise being performed. High frequency and high intensity exercise will generally be performed for shorter time periods. Low intensity exercise can be performed for longer periods. Exercise duration is also dependent upon the time available for exercise. If an individual only has 15 minutes available for exercise in a given day, 15 minutes will be the duration of the exercise period. Most experts recommend a minimum of 30 minutes per day to maintain health.

Summary

The FIT principle is a tool used by trainers to help individuals and athletes develop training programs to reach their goals. Trainers develop exercise programs based on frequency, intensity, and the amount of time a person should exercise. By varying the frequency, intensity, and time of the exercises performed, individuals and athletes can achieve very different goals for their bodies, health, and fitness levels using exercise. Each of the three components of the FIT principle is related to the others and must be considered in conjunction with the others when developing an exercise plan. High intensity or long duration exercise performed too frequently will result in weakening of the muscles, loss of muscle mass, and damage to the ligaments and tendons. Athletes vary their exercise plan each day to avoid overtraining injuries. Exercise intensity asks the question, "How hard are you working?" High intensity aerobic exercise increases the heart rate and is usually measured using a heart rate monitor. The intensity of strength training is generally determined using the amount of weight, the number of sets, and the number of repetitions within each set. High frequency and high intensity exercise will generally be performed for shorter time periods. Low intensity exercise can be performed for longer periods. Exercise duration is also dependent upon the time available for exercise.

Concept Reinforcement

1. What is the FIT principle?

2. Why is frequency of exercise important?

3. How is the intensity of an aerobic workout determined?

Section 2.12 – Power, Strength, and Endurance

Section Objectives

- Define power and what principles make a movement powerful
- Explain the differences between strength and endurance training

Power

When discussing physical performance under exercise, **power** refers to the speed with which strength can be applied to move a **sub maximal load**. For example, moving a 50 lb weight 3 ft in 1 second is more powerful than moving a 50 lb weight 3 ft in 3 seconds, even though both efforts require the same amount of strength, the ability to lift 50 lbs. The vertical leap test is typically used to assess athletic power. Power is measured in

Watts (W) = Force (in Newtons) × distance (in meters) ÷ time (in seconds).

Strength is the force a muscle can exert against resistance, measured in Newtons (N). Powerful movements are explosive, they happen very rapidly and with great strength. Think of linemen in a football game. When the ball is snapped, they quickly collide with one another, using their utmost strength to move each other out of position and make a play.

> A **sub-maximal load** is any weight that is less than the **one rep max** for an individual.
>
> The **one rep max** is the maximum amount of weight an individual can lift one time.

Principles of powerful movement

Power is a function of speed and strength. Athletes use strength training with weights to increase muscular strength. However, slow weightlifting movements will only increase strength. Movements must be made quickly. To this end, athletes often train using a method known as **plyometrics**. Plyometrics are exercises that are performed rapidly and explosively. The involve leaping, pushing off of surfaces with the hands, or both. Athletes may also incorporate speed training elements into their workout regimens. Sprinting, running stairs, and punching a speed bag help increase the speed with which movements can be made. The result is that the neuromuscular signaling time is reduced and movements can be made more quickly.

Power can be affected by the athlete's familiarity with the movement. The more practiced a movement is, the more quickly the athlete can perform it and the more powerful it is. Athletes practice specific techniques until they are performed without thought.

Strength Versus Endurance

Endurance is different from strength. **Endurance** is the ability of the muscle to contact over long periods of time. **Strength** is the force a muscle can exert against resistance. Endurance training focuses on low to moderate intensity exercises performed for long periods of time. Strength training focuses on high intensity exercises performed over short time frames. Endurance training improves the efficiency of the muscle. In so doing, the muscle may actually *decrease* in both size and strength. Endurance training includes improvements in the efficiency of the cardiovascular system to carry oxygen and nutrients to the muscles and remove waste products. Strength training focuses on increasing the diameter of the muscles, increasing the number of **myofilaments** in the muscle, and the density of the connective tissue surrounding the muscles. Strength training improves the anaerobic capabilities of the muscles.

> **Myofilaments** are the proteins inside the muscle cells of the skeletal muscle that are responsible for muscle contraction.

Endurance training typically uses the weight of the body, and involves running, cycling, or swimming as training methods. Strength training utilizes resistance with weights or elastic bands.

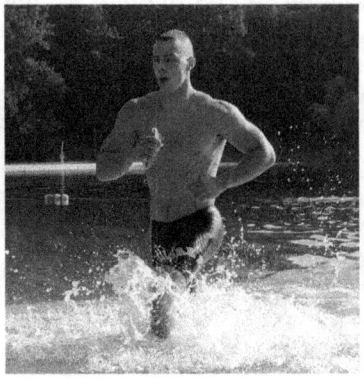

Lance Corporal Anthony M. Madonia emerges from the water during the swimming portion of the triathlon. Marines and Sailors of Marine Security Company and the Naval Support Facility in Thurmont, Maryland, participated in the Catoctin Mountain Triathlon July 20, 2005.
Image courtesy of the U.S. Marine Corps. Triathlons are examples of endurance events.

Summary

When discussing physical performance under exercise, power refers to the speed with which strength can be applied to move a sub maximal load. Power is measured in Watts (W) = Force (in Newtons) x distance (in meters) ÷ time (in seconds). Powerful movements are explosive, they happen very rapidly and with great strength. Athletes use strength training with weights, plyometrics, and speed training elements in their workout regimens to increase power. The result is that the neuromuscular signaling time is reduced and movements can be made more quickly. Power can be affected by the athlete's familiarity with the movement. The more practiced a movement is, the more quickly the athlete can perform it and the more powerful it is. Endurance is the ability of the muscle to contact over long periods of time. Endurance training focuses on low to moderate intensity exercises performed for long periods of time to improve the efficiency of the muscle. Endurance training includes improvements in the efficiency of the cardiovascular system to carry oxygen and nutrients to the muscles and remove waste products. Strength is the force a muscle can exert against resistance. Strength training focuses on high intensity exercises performed over short time frames to increase the diameter of the muscles, the number of myofilaments in the muscle, and the density of the connective tissue surrounding the muscles. Strength training improves the anaerobic capabilities of the muscles.

Concept Reinforcements

1. Explain how power is calculated and give an example.

2. List the three training methods athletes use to increase their power and how this training is effective.

3. Describe the difference between strength and endurance training.

Section 2.13 – Interval Training: Aerobic and Anaerobic Conditioning

Section Objective

- Define aerobic conditioning, anaerobic conditioning, and interval training and discuss their effects on fitness level

Aerobic Conditioning

Aerobic conditioning is physical training which improves the body's ability to take in, distribute, and use oxygen during exercise. Aerobic conditioning improves the ability of the heart to pump blood, enhances blood delivery to the muscles, and improves the efficiency with which the muscles convert **glucose**, the sugar used by the cells to make energy, into **ATP**, adenosine triphosphate, the energy source used in cellular metabolism. Aerobic conditioning programs involve low to moderate intensity exercise performed over long periods of time. Running, cycling, and swimming are commonly used exercises that build aerobic capacity. Rowing is a particularly good aerobic exercise. However, circuit training with weights is also an effective aerobic workout. Aerobic conditioning involves the use of **overload** and **progression**. Overload means that the body must work beyond its normal capability in order to improve its condition. Progression, an increase in the intensity of the work done, continues to improve performance once the body becomes comfortable at the new intensity.

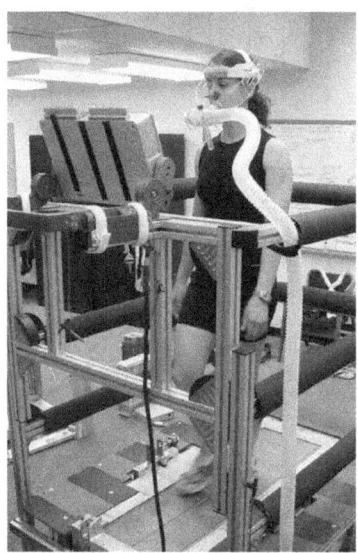

This image depicts Leah Stroud, an Exercise Lab assistant, exercising on Treadmill with Vibration Isolation and Stabilization (TVIS) at the JSC Exercise Laboratory while metabolic rate was measured. Photo courtesy of NASA.

To stimulate aerobic conditioning, the heart must beat at between 75 and 80% of its maximum rate. The maximum heart rate is calculated by subtracting the athlete's age from 220. For a 15 year old athlete, aerobic conditioning will be stimulated when the heart rate is maintained at (220-15) x 75% or 80%, or 154 to 164 beats per minute for 10 to 30 minutes. As long as the heart rate is maintained within the target zone, regardless of the exercise performed, aerobic conditioning is improved. Over time, the athlete will have to work with greater intensity to reach the target heart rate because of improvements in aerobic fitness.

Anaerobic Conditioning

When the body is required to perform at an intensity level beyond that which can be sustained by aerobic metabolism, it shifts energy production to anaerobic processes. The athlete is said to be in **oxygen debt**, and the oxygen debt will be repaid when the exercise intensity decreases. Anaerobic metabolism is much less efficient in converting glucose into ATP and creates lactic acid as a by-product. Lactic acid will be metabolized into energy by the muscles when exercise intensity decreases and sufficient oxygen is again available. Anaerobic conditioning involves overload and progression, just as aerobic conditioning does. However, the overload used during anaerobic conditioning will be greater in order to force the body into oxygen debt. This will stimulate improvement in the muscles' anaerobic metabolic system. It will also improve the muscles' ability to recover from oxygen debt. Interval training is the best method to improve anaerobic conditioning.

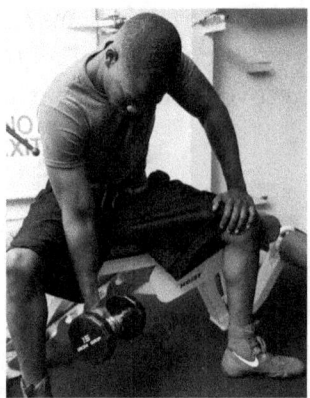

Anaerobic training improves muscle strength and recovery from oxygen debt.

Interval Training

Interval training involves short bursts of high intensity exercise interspersed between longer periods of low intensity aerobic exercise. Because of its nature, high intensity training cannot be performed over long periods of time. By training in short bursts of high intensity training, the body is placed into oxygen debt, and it must adapt itself to function in the anaerobic state and recover from it. Continuing to exercise at a lower intensity, for example walking, helps the body recover. Interval training generally uses ratios of high intensity exercise to rest of 1:4 to 1:1. For example, after a 100 meter sprint that takes 12 seconds, the athlete should rest for 48 seconds, then run the next 100 m sprint (1:4). As fitness improves, the amount of rest can be reduced. A fit athlete might run 100 m in 12 seconds, then rest 12 seconds (1:1) before sprinting the next 100 m. The "rested" heart rate during interval training should be approximately 70% of the maximum heart rate. While in the intense phase of the interval, the heart rate should be approximately 90% of maximum.

Interval training improves the body's ability to recover from anaerobic activity, improves anaerobic metabolism, and increases strength. By adding an aerobic workout on alternating days, the body develops a higher anaerobic threshold. The combination of aerobic and interval training significantly boost fitness by improving the body's ability to function at a higher intensity for longer periods and to recover faster.

Summary

Aerobic conditioning is physical training which improves the body's ability to take in, distribute, and use oxygen during exercise. Aerobic conditioning improves the ability of the heart to pump blood, enhances blood delivery to the muscles, and improves the efficiency with which the muscles convert glucose into ATP. Aerobic conditioning programs involve low to moderate intensity exercise performed over long periods of time. The body shifts energy production to anaerobic processes when it is required to perform at an intensity level beyond that which can be sustained by aerobic metabolism. The athlete enters oxygen debt, which will be repaid when the exercise intensity decreases. Anaerobic metabolism is less efficient in converting glucose into ATP and creates lactic acid as a by-product. Interval training involves short bursts of high intensity exercise interspersed between longer periods of low intensity aerobic exercise. By training in short bursts of high intensity training, the body is placed into oxygen debt, and it must adapt itself to function in the anaerobic state and recover from it. The combination of aerobic and interval training significantly boost fitness by improving the body's ability to function at a higher intensity for longer periods and to recover faster.

Concept Reinforcement

1. What is aerobic conditioning?

2. What is anaerobic conditioning?

3. How does interval training improve fitness?

Section 2.14 – Sets and Repetitions

Section Objective

- Define sets and repetitions and describe how they are used in sports training

Sets and Repetitions

A **repetition**, or **rep**, is a single exercise movement from start to finish. A **set** is a group of repetitions. Sets and repetitions are the means of dividing up exercise into manageable portions which can then be tailored into a training program. They also permit athletes and trainers to adjust the intensity of a workout. For example, a biceps curl is performed by starting with a weight held in the hand with the arm hanging down at the side. The weight is then lifted by bending the arm at the elbow to raise the weight to the top of the shoulder. The weight is finally lowered in a controlled motion to the starting point. The entire procedure is a single repetition. A single repetition is not enough to exercise a muscle. Instead, athletes perform several repetitions of the same exercise at a time in sets. Performing ten repetitions of a biceps curl in a row would be one set of ten reps. A set is followed by a period of rest to allow the muscle to clear its oxygen debt and be ready for the next set. There is no specific number of repetitions that is required to make a set. The number of reps in a set depends upon the goals of the athlete.

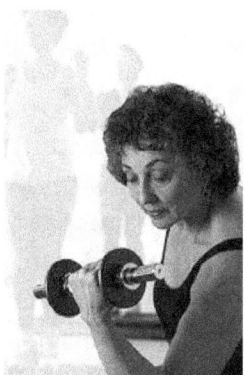

A single repetition of a biceps curl is performed by starting with a weight held in the hand with the arm hanging down at the side. The weight is then lifted by bending the arm at the elbow to raise the weight to the top of the shoulder. The weight is finally lowered in a controlled motion to the starting point.
Image courtesy of the Centers for Disease Control

Using Sets and Reps in Training

The goals of athletes training in different sports are dependent upon the sport and the position played. Linemen on a football team require tremendous strength and power. Forwards on a soccer team must be fast and must possess exceptional endurance. Each athlete will train using weights, but they will train differently. By varying the number of reps and sets, athletes can achieve very different goals using the same exercises.

To train for strength, an athlete will use heavy weights, low reps, and low to moderate numbers of sets. A typical strength routine would utilize weight the athlete is capable of lifting for no more than six reps in a set, with from three to six sets. Once the athlete can perform six reps for most or all of his sets, the weight should be increased.

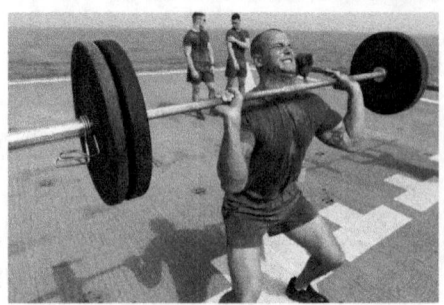

Utilization of heavy weights, low reps, and low to moderate numbers of sets increases strength.

Endurance training typically utilizes lighter weights and higher reps and sets. Athletes may perform five or six sets of ten to twelve reps. Sets and reps can also be counted during interval training. Athletes may sprint 100 m five times, followed by a set of 50 m sprints, followed by a set of 10 m sprints.

Training for power typically utilizes intermediate weight and intermediate sets and reps. Athletes may use three to five sets of six to eight reps. An athlete would increase the weight she uses only after reaching eight reps in all, or nearly all of her sets.

Summary

A repetition, or rep, is a single exercise movement from start to finish. A set is a group of repetitions. Sets and repetitions are the means of dividing up exercise into manageable portions which can then be tailored into a training program. They also permit athletes and trainers to adjust the intensity of a workout. A set is followed by a period of rest to allow the muscle to clear its oxygen debt and be ready for the next set. There is no specific number of repetitions that is required to make a set. The number of reps in a set depends upon the goals of the athlete. By varying the number of reps and sets, athletes can achieve very different goals using the same exercises. To train for strength, an athlete will use heavy weights, low reps, and low to moderate numbers of sets. Endurance training typically utilizes lighter weights and higher reps and sets. Training for power typically utilizes intermediate weight and intermediate sets and reps.

Concept Reinforcement

1. Describe the difference between a set and a rep.

2. How can the same exercise create different results for different athletes?

3. Describe the difference between a strength routine and an endurance routine.

Section 2.15 – Thibaudeau's Six Training Programs

Section Objective

- List Thibaudeau's 6 types of training programs and describe how each is unique

Christian Thibaudeau is a Canadian Olympic weightlifter, bodybuilder, athletic coach, and trainer. He is a regular contributor to a number of fitness and bodybuilding magazines, graduated with a M.Sc. in exercise physiology, and has written several books on physical training.

Force Production

Thibaudeau notes that **force** and **strength** are two different concepts which are frequently confused, and the terms are often used interchangeably. **Force** is the result of tension produced by muscle to move mass. **Strength** is the ability to produce force during muscular contraction. The difference is subtle, but important; force must be produced, strength is the ability to produce that force. **Force** equals mass times acceleration. In order to move a mass, the athlete must first generate enough force to overcome the **inertia** of the object, its weight. Then she must accelerate the mass. How rapidly she moves that mass is a function of her ability to generate force, her strength. By increasing the speed with which she can accelerate the mass, she can increase her strength without increasing the weight she must move. Any athletic training program should focus on improving the athlete's **force production** rather than just strength.

Training Methods

Thibaudeau identified six training programs that can be used to increase an athlete's force production. The methods trainers can use to improve an athlete's performance range from very rapid movement with light weights to very slow movements with very heavy weights. Each method will improve an athlete's force production, but they will do so using different proportions of sheer muscular strength to acceleration of the mass. The first three methods discussed below are speed dominant programs. They use lighter weights, create **power** (the rapid application of strength), and develop readily transferable force production capacity for most sports. The last three methods discussed below are strength dominant programs. They use heavier weights, increase muscle mass and tendon strength, and serve as the foundation for power and other physical characteristics.

Ballistic Method

Acceleration is the dominant component of the Ballistic method of training. The ballistic method involves "throwing" the weight, hence the name ballistic. The weight thrown may be a medicine ball or the athlete's own body weight. Exercises include plyometrics (exercises performed explosively using the weight of the body or light weights), loaded absorption drills, and leaping drills. The intensity of the exercises can vary from low intensity leaps to extremely high weighted jumping and landing drills. Low impact ballistic drills can actually be used as warm-ups before beginning other training programs. High intensity drills can be damaging if used too frequently. Ballistic training impacts the nervous system, causing more muscle fibers to be activated more rapidly.

Speed-Strength Method

The Speed-strength method is dominated by acceleration as well. The method utilizes light weights, and typically involves sports-related movements. Ankle and wrist weights or weighted shoes or skates increase the force required to perform sports movements. A potential drawback to this kind of training is that athletes may alter their technique to compensate for the additional weight. When the weights are removed during competition, the adaptation may detract from optimum performance or create errors that can lead to falls and injury. Care must be taken by trainers to avoid this potential eventuality.

Strength-Speed Method

Acceleration and strength are equally important in the Strength-speed method. Thibaudeau recommends that at least 30% of an athlete's workout should utilize Strength-speed techniques. Rapid acceleration of moderate to heavy mass is the goal of this method. Athletes may use between 55 and 80% of their maximum lift weight in these exercises, and lift the weight as rapidly as possible. Olympic style lifts such as the snatch and the clean and press are commonly used to accomplish the goals of the Strength-speed method. However, the bench press, squat, and sports-related moves may be used as well. Care must be taken when performing Olympic style lifts because of the complexity of the movements. Athletes should be completely familiar with the lift before increasing from moderate to heavy weights.

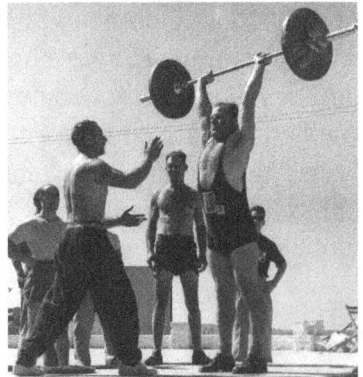

An Olympic style lift utilizes both strength and acceleration to lift moderate to heavy weights rapidly.

Controlled Repetition Method

The Controlled repetition method is the classic bodybuilding method of heavy weights and isolation of specific muscle groups, coupled with controlled, relatively slow movements. These movements can create **hypertrophy**, increase in size, of muscles. However, it does little to increase strength and power. In fact, extremely large muscles can impede athletic performance. Hypertrophy of muscles can be caused by increases in non-contractile components of muscle. In this case, even though the muscle is larger, strength does not change. This method is best used to strengthen trouble spots for specific athletes or to increase the strength of tendons and other connective tissue in areas such as the rotator cuff.

Maximal Method

The Maximal method combines maximum weight lifting, eccentric exercises, and isometric exercises to rapidly increase muscular strength. **Maximum weight lifting** involves lifting masses of 85 to 100% of the athlete's maximum weight. **Eccentric exercises** utilize loads of 90 to 100% of the athlete's maximum weight. However instead of lifting the weight as would normally be done, the movement is performed in reverse; the load is lowered as slowly as possible, then raised with assistance if needed. **Isometric exercises** involve exerting maximum effort to move an immovable object. The Maximal method emphasizes low repetitions, 2-6, and few sets, 2-5. The Maximal method maximizes strength gains, but if overused can lead to loss of strength due to overtraining of the muscles.

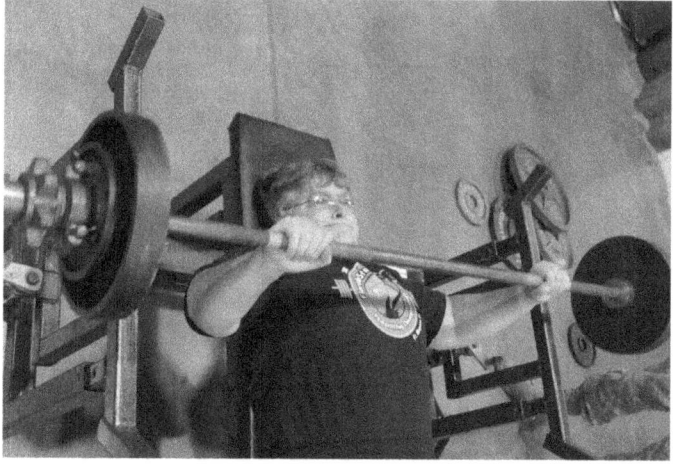

Carol Adams is a disabled Army veteran who competes in power lifting events.

Supra-Maximal Method

The Supra-maximal method must be used with extreme care. The athlete will be lifting loads in excess of his maximum capability. This method can lead to dramatic gains in strength and break through plateaus, or it can result in injury and setbacks. Supra-maximal loads are lifted eccentrically, the athlete uses improper form to get past the sticking point, or the athlete does not use a complete range of motion for the exercise. Athletes should perform only a very few reps using this method, and it should be used infrequently.

Summary

Thibaudeau notes that force is the result of tension produced by muscle to move mass while strength is the ability to produce force during muscular contraction. Force equals mass times acceleration. In order to move a mass, the athlete must first generate enough force to overcome the inertia of the object, its weight. Then she must accelerate the mass. How rapidly she moves that mass is a function of her ability to generate force, her strength. By increasing the speed with which she can accelerate the mass, she can increase her strength without increasing the weight she must move. Any athletic training program should focus on improving the athlete's force production rather than just strength. Thibaudeau identified six training programs that can be used to increase an athlete's force production. Acceleration is the dominant component of the Ballistic method of training. The ballistic method involves "throwing" the weight, hence the name ballistic. Exercises include throwing a medicine ball, plyometrics, loaded absorption drills, and leaping drills. The Speed-strength method is dominated by acceleration as well. The method utilizes light weights, and typically involves sports-related movements. Ankle and wrist weights or weighted shoes or skates increase the force required to perform sports movements. Acceleration and strength are equally important in the Strength-speed method. Rapid acceleration of moderate to heavy mass is the goal of this method. The Controlled repetition method is the classic bodybuilding method of heavy weights and isolation of specific muscle groups, coupled with controlled, relatively slow movements. These movements can create hypertrophy of muscles, but may not increase strength and power. The Maximal method combines maximum weight lifting, eccentric exercises, and isometric exercises to rapidly increase muscular strength. The Maximal method maximizes strength gains, but if overused can lead to loss of strength due to overtraining of the muscles. The Supra-maximal method must be used with extreme care. The athlete will be lifting loads in excess of his maximum capability. This method can lead to dramatic gains in strength and break through plateaus, or it can result in injury and setbacks.

Concept Reinforcement

1. List and briefly describe Thibaudeau's six training methods.

2. Explain the concept of force production.

3. How is it possible for an athlete to lift more than her maximal weight?

Unit Three

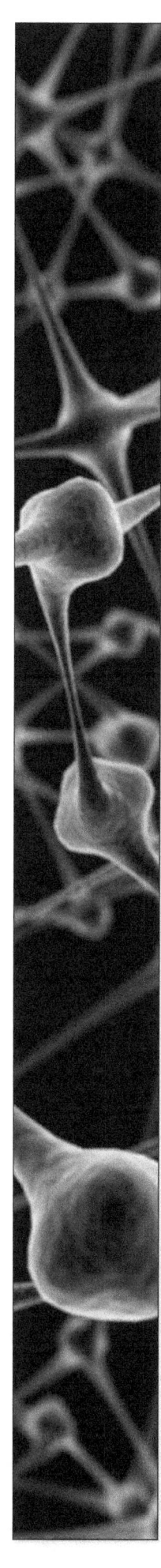

Section 3.1 – Brain Injuries   150

Section 3.2 – Spinal Cord Injuries   155

Section 3.3 – Assessment and Treatment of Spinal Cord Injuries   159

Section 3.4 – The Shoulder and Shoulder Injuries   163

Section 3.5 – The Elbow and Elbow Injuries   167

Section 3.6 – The Body's Core   169

Section 3.7 – The Wrist   173

Section 3.8 – The Hand   177

Section 3.9 – The Spinal Column   181

Section 3.10 – The Hip   187

Section 3.11 – Structure of the Knee   189

Section 3.12 – Knee Injuries   191

Section 3.13 – The Ankle and Ankle Injuries   193

Section 3.14 – The Foot and Foot Injuries   197

Section 3.15 – Osteoarthritis   201

Section 3.1 – Brain Injuries

Section Objectives

- Describe the difference between focal and diffuse traumatic brain injuries
- Define the term concussion and explain the mechanism that causes a concussion

Brain Injuries

Brain injuries are life-threatening and should always be taken seriously. Brain injuries can be of several types, but most are either due to trauma to the brain caused by a blow or to loss of oxygen from a stroke or breathing stoppage. Concussions are a specific type of traumatic brain injury. In the following discussion the causes and effects of brain trauma will be examined.

Traumatic Brain Injury

Traumatic brain injury is direct damage to the brain caused by an external force. There are closed skull and open skull traumatic injuries. **Open skull injuries** occur when an object breaks the skull and damages the brain by pushing part of the skull into the brain, or when the object itself penetrates to the brain and causes damage. These types of injuries are common in vehicular accidents, sports, falls, and violent crime. **Closed skull injuries** occur when the head is rapidly accelerated or decelerated. The brain moves independently of the skull, and can crash into the skull if the head moves too rapidly. These injuries are common in vehicular crashes, shaken baby syndrome, falls, and crime. For example, a **coup-countre coup** injury to the brain occurs in rear-end automotive crashes when the head snaps backwards. The brain is slammed into the front of the skull as the head snaps back. The brain then bounces backward as the head rebounds forward, and the rear of the brain impacts with the back of the skull.

A **focal brain injury** is an injury to the brain that is limited to a specific area of the brain. There is a focal point where the injury occurred and the damage was done. Focal brain injuries are typically caused by a blow to the head, criminal assault, or a bullet. Focal brain injuries can be either open or closed skull. The symptoms of a focal brain injury are directly related to the region of the brain where the injury occurred. If the hearing centers of the brain are damaged, hearing will be impaired. If the damage is done to the memory centers of the brain, memory will be affected.

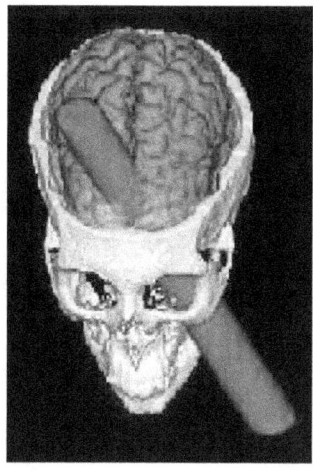

This computer-generated graphic shows how, in 1848, a 3-foot long, pointed rod penetrated the skull of Phineas Gage, a railway construction foreman. The rod entered at the top of his head, passed through his brain, and exited his skull by his temple. Gage survived the accident but suffered lasting personality and behavioral problems.

A **diffuse brain injury** is an injury to the brain that affects most or all of the brain with no specific site of tissue damage. Diffuse brain injuries are often the result of disease or **vascular disruption**, damage to or stoppage of the circulation of blood. The damage to the brain in diffuse brain injuries occurs at the cellular level and is very difficult to diagnose. The chance of survival after diffuse brain injury is very low. There are four types of diffuse brain injury:

- Diffuse vascular injury

- Diffuse swelling

- Diffuse hypoxic/anoxic/ischemic injury

- Diffuse axonal injury

Diffuse vascular injury is commonly the result of a major head trauma and is characterized by numerous small hemorrhages within the brain. Patients usually die within 24 hours. **Diffuse swelling** is caused by **edema** in the brain, leakage of fluid into the brain. Diffuse swelling usually occurs as the result of a traumatic injury to the head. Edema raises the pressure in the brain and presses the brain against the membranes which surround and protect it. The brain can be **herniated**, forced through some of these membranes. It also presses strongly against the skull. When the pressure in the skull rises above 60 mm Hg the patient dies. Diffuse **hypoxic/anoxic/ischemic injury** is caused by disruption of the flow of blood to the brain. This can occur as a result of massive trauma to the body with concurrent loss of blood pressure, heart attack, or extremely high **intracranial pressure**, pressure within the skull, which can prevent blood from entering the brain. **Diffuse axonal injury** is often the result of head trauma that results in shearing of the axons. The axons are the neural projections from the neural cell body to the target tissue. The axons can either be shorn as a result of the injury, or secondarily a few hours after the injury. Diffuse axonal injury is diagnosed **post-mortem**, or after death.

Concussion

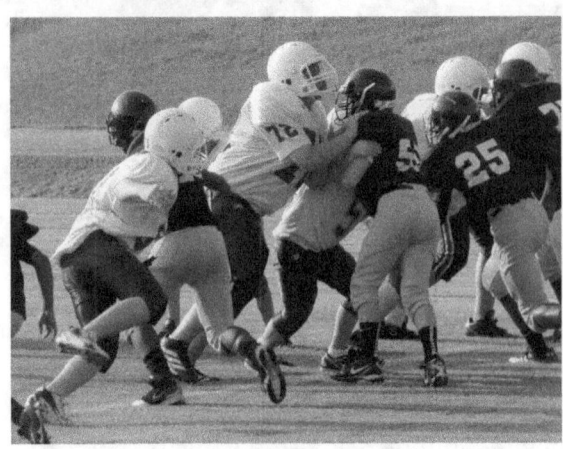

Concussions are increasing among high school students who participate in sports. Recovery time for high school athletes who suffer from a concussion are longer than for college athletes.

A **concussion** is a brain injury that results from a blow to the head, violent shaking of the head, gunshots, and whiplash injuries. Concussions are the mildest form of brain injury, but are nonetheless very serious. Concussions are difficult to diagnose. They may or may not involve short term (less than 20 minutes) loss of consciousness. The patient may report feeling dazed or stunned. A concussion may or may not be visible on a CAT scan. Skull fracture, bleeding in the brain, and brain swelling may or may not be present. Diffuse axonal injury is a possible secondary injury resulting from a concussion that may not occur for hours after the injury. Recall that diffuse axonal injury often causes death. For this reason, all concussions should be taken very seriously. Blood clots may also form in the vasculature of the brain and cause strokes. Concussions may require months or years to fully heal.

Summary

Brain injuries can be of several types, but most are either due to trauma to the brain caused by a blow or to loss of oxygen from a stroke or breathing stoppage. Traumatic brain injury is direct damage to the brain caused by an external force. There are closed skull and open skull traumatic injuries. Open skull injuries occur when an object breaks the skull and damages the brain. Closed skull injuries occur when the head is rapidly accelerated or decelerated. The brain moves independently of the skull, and can crash into the skull if the head moves too rapidly. A focal brain injury is an injury to the brain that is limited to a specific area of the brain, and can be either open or closed skull. The symptoms of a focal brain injury are directly related to the region of the brain where the injury occurred. A diffuse brain injury is an injury to the brain that affects most or all of the brain with no specific site of tissue damage. The damage to the brain in diffuse brain injuries occurs at the cellular level and is very difficult to diagnose. The chance of survival after diffuse brain injury is very low. There are four types of diffuse brain injury: diffuse vascular injury, diffuse swelling, diffuse hypoxic/anoxic/ischemic injury, and diffuse axonal injury. Concussions are the mildest form of brain injury, but are nonetheless very serious. Concussions are difficult to diagnose. Diffuse axonal injury is a possible secondary injury resulting from a concussion that may not occur for hours after the injury. Blood clots may also form in the vasculature of the brain and cause strokes. Concussions may require months or years to fully heal.

Concept Reinforcement

1. Describe a focal brain injury.
2. Describe the four types of diffuse brain injuries.
3. Describe a concussion.

Section 3.2 – Spinal Cord Injuries

Section Objectives

- Discuss various types of spinal cord injuries and how they affect body functioning
- Define axial load and how it contributes to cervical spinal cord injury

Spinal Cord Injuries

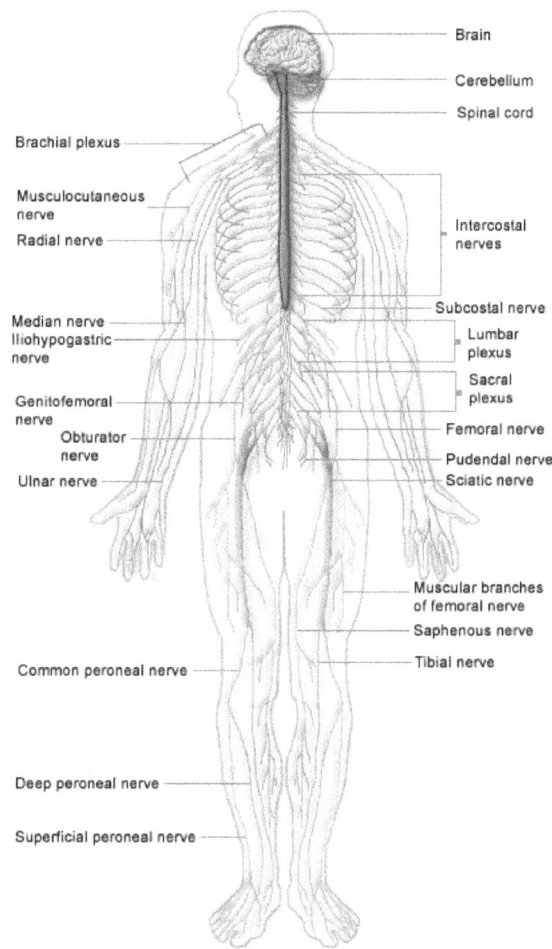

In the United States, there are over 450,000 people who live with spinal cord injuries. Approximately 10,000 new cases occur each year, and 82% of those cases will be in males between the ages of 16 and 30. Spinal cord injuries vary significantly in their effects, depending upon where the injury occurs and the severity of the injury. Spinal cord injuries can be **complete** or **incomplete**. Complete spinal cord injuries result in complete loss of sensation and control on both sides of the body below the injury. Incomplete spinal cord injuries permit some level of sensation and control below the injury. Advances in treatments for spinal cord injuries have increased the occurrence of incomplete spinal cord injuries while decreasing the incidence of complete spinal cord injuries. Spinal cord injuries are designated C1-C8, T1-T12, L1-L5, and S1-S5.

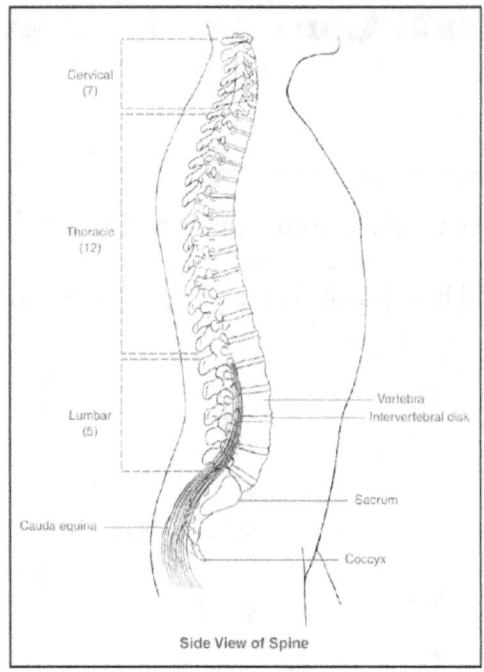
Side View of Spine

C1-C8 injuries occur in the **cervical vertebrae**, or in the neck region, and affect the entire body. Quadriplegia, paralysis of all of the limbs is the result of damage above C5. Injuries above C4 may require the patient to use a ventilator to breathe. Some control of the biceps and shoulders may occur for C5 injuries. Injuries at C6 can leave some control of the wrists, but not the hands. Injuries below C7 or T1 do not usually prevent full control of the arms and hands.

Injuries to the **thoracic vertebrae** (T1-T12), those of the upper to middle back, result in paraplegia. Patients are unable to control the body below the point of injury. T1-T8 injuries result in good hand control, but patients will have difficulty sitting upright because of the loss of control over the abdominal and lower back muscles. Patients with injuries below T9 can usually sit with good posture.

Injuries to the **lumbar vertebrae** (L1-L5), or lower back, affect the hips and legs. Injuries nearer L5 result in better control over the hips and legs, while injuries closer to L1 result in poor leg and hip control.

Injuries to the **sacral vertebrae** (S1-S5), those found below the hip bone, may affect bowel, bladder, and sexual function.

Spinal cord injuries can also cause loss of blood pressure, breathing, bladder, and bowel control, loss of the ability to sweat below the injury, sexual dysfunction, and chronic pain.

Axial Load and Cervical Injuries

The first two vertebrae beneath the skull are called the atlas (C1) and the axis (C2). **Axial loading** refers to placing a load on the second vertebra of the spinal column, the **axis**, usually as a result of a blow to the top of the head. These injuries are most common in young athletes, especially in football, diving, rugby, and gymnastics. Axial loading occurs when the spine is straightened by lowering the head slightly. This position prevents the ligaments, tendons, and muscles from absorbing the impact and transmits the force to the vertebra. The vertebra can be crushed, or it can slide forward, backward or laterally to shear the spinal cord. In football, the form of tackling called "spearing", in which the tackler leads with the crown of the helmet, straightens the vertebrae and greatly increases the danger of cervical injury due to axial loading. Outlawing of the practice dramatically lowered the incidence of cervical injuries due to axial loading in football players. Similarly in diving, the head is lowered and if the head strikes an object below the surface of the water, cervical injury can occur.

Summary

In the United States, there are over 450,000 people who live with spinal cord injuries. Approximately 10,000 new cases occur each year. Sixteen to thirty year old males account for 82% of spinal cord injury cases. Spinal cord injuries can be complete, resulting in complete loss of sensation and control on both sides of the body below the injury, or incomplete, permitting some level of sensation and control below the injury. C1-C8 injuries occur in the cervical vertebrae, or in the neck region, and affect the entire body.

Injuries to the thoracic vertebrae (T1-T12), those of the upper to middle back, result in paraplegia. Injuries to the lumbar vertebrae (L1-L5), or lower back, affect the hips and legs. Injuries to the sacral vertebrae (S1-S5), those found below the hip bone, may affect bowel, bladder, and sexual function. Spinal cord injuries can also cause loss of blood pressure, breathing, bladder, and bowel control, loss of the ability to sweat below the injury, sexual dysfunction, and chronic pain. Axial loading refers to placing a load on the second vertebra of the spinal column, the axis, usually as a result of a blow to the top of the head. These injuries are most common in young athletes, especially in football, diving, rugby, and gymnastics. Axial loading occurs when the spine is straightened by lowering the head slightly. This position prevents the ligaments, tendons, and muscles from absorbing the impact and transmits the force to the vertebra. The vertebra can be crushed, or it can slide forward, backward or laterally to shear the spinal cord.

Concept Reinforcement

1. Compare complete and incomplete spinal cord injuries.

2. List the four levels at which spinal cord injuries can occur and explain how the level of the injury affects the body.

3. Explain axial loading injury and why it is crucial to young athletes.

Section 3.3 – Assessment and Treatment of Spinal Cord Injuries

Section Objectives

- Describe the assessment and current treatments for spinal cord injuries

- Assessment and treatment of spinal cord injuries

First-Responder Actions

Spinal cord injuries are usually the result of a major trauma and are often accompanied by a number of other significant injuries. Spinal cord injuries can result in life-threatening secondary conditions such as loss of blood pressure and inability to breathe. Emergency responders to spinal cord injury must remember **the ABC's of emergency medicine**: Airway, Breathing, Circulation. If the patient is not breathing because of a blocked airway or for some other reason, death will soon follow and the spinal injury is a secondary concern. Likewise, if the patient's heart is not beating or if the patient is suffering from significant blood loss and loss of blood pressure, death is imminent. While care should be taken to avoid exacerbating the spinal injury, the patient's life is the paramount concern. Once the patient is breathing and blood is circulating properly, the spine should be completely immobilized. The neck should be secured with a cervical hard collar and the patient should be securely immobilized on a hard backboard for transportation to the hospital.

Assessment of Spinal Cord Injury

Once the patient arrives at the hospital, the doctor should repeat the ABC's of emergency medicine. Poor or no respiration may indicate a high cervical spinal cord injury. The patient should be removed from the backboard as quickly as possible to prevent pain. The doctor should then collect a complete **history** of the injury. In other words, she should ask the patient to describe what happened, any signs or symptoms, and whether there are any sensory or motor deficits. The next step will be to complete a neurological assessment. A **neurological assessment** determines the patient's level of consciousness (alert to unconscious), **mentation** (ability to process thoughts), pupil dilation, motor function (ability to move), sensory responses (responsiveness to soft, sharp, cold, hot, and vibrating objects), and reflex responses (especially to deep tendon reflexes). The level of response will help the doctor gauge whether the spinal cord injury is incomplete, affecting one side or allowing some level of function, or complete, both sides of the body are unable to move or sense stimuli. She will be able to determine the likely location of the injury based on the areas of the body that are unresponsive. The physical examination is followed by either X-rays or CT scans of the spine. In the event damage to the spinal cord without concurrent damage to the vertebrae is suspected, a MRI should be conducted to detect the damage to the soft tissues of the spinal cord.

Treatment of Spinal Cord Injuries

During the examination and afterward, it is not uncommon for spinal cord injury patients to be in great pain. The doctor should provide **analgesic medications**, pain relievers, to reduce the pain and ease the exam procedure. The National Acute Spinal Cord Injury Studies (NASCIS) II and III have concluded that patients with spinal cord injuries should be treated with high doses of **methylprednisolone** within 8 hours of injury. Methylprednisolone is a synthetic **corticosteroid**, a steroid that mimics those produced by the adrenal gland. Corticosteroids reduce inflammation and suppress the immune system. Patients receiving methylprednisolone within 8 hours of injury exhibit better function and less injury than patients who do not receive methylprednisolone. New studies are calling the current practice into question, but it is still a recommended therapy for spinal cord injury.

The skin of patients suffering from spinal cord injuries is very prone to **pressure necrosis**, death of the tissue due to pressure applied to the tissue. Belts, keys, wallets, and other hard objects should be removed from the patient, and portions of the body that will be in contact with surfaces should be padded. Patients should be turned ever 1-2 hours to limit the likelihood of pressure necrosis.

Patients with spinal cord injuries are subject to numerous complications as a result of their injury. Spinal cord injury patients must be watched carefully for lung problems and poor or no breathing. **Hypothermia**, low body temperature, is another threatening complication. Pneumonia and urinary tract infections are common. Spinal cord patients with complete injuries typically died within a year because of pneumonia and urinary tract infections up until the 1990's when antibiotics were more commonly prescribed.

After the initial hospitalization period, the patient will require extensive physical and occupational therapy. However, 90% of spinal cord injury patients return home and regain their independence.

At the time of this writing, the US Food and Drug Administration (FDA) has approved a phase I clinical trial to use stem cells to treat crush injury patients with thoracic spinal cord injuries. While a therapy is still a long way off, there is some hope that in the future, spinal cord injury patients will be able to regain most if not all of their previous level of function.

Summary

Spinal cord injuries are usually the result of a major trauma and are often accompanied by a number of other significant injuries. Emergency responders to spinal cord injury must remember the ABC's of emergency medicine: Airway, Breathing, Circulation. The spine should be completely immobilized; the neck should be secured with a cervical hard collar and the patient should be securely immobilized on a hard backboard for transportation to the hospital. The doctor should collect a complete history of the injury and complete a neurological assessment, followed by X-rays, CT scans, or MRI of the spine. The doctor should provide analgesic medications and high doses of methylprednisolone within 8 hours of injury. Belts, keys, wallets, and other hard objects should be removed from the patient, and portions of the body that will be in contact with surfaces should be padded. Patients should be turned ever 1-2 hours to limit the likelihood of pressure necrosis. Spinal cord injury patients must be watched carefully for lung problems and poor or no breathing, hypothermia, pneumonia, and urinary tract infections. The patient will require extensive physical and occupational therapy, but 90% of spinal cord injury patients return home and regain their independence. At the time of this writing, the US Food and Drug Administration (FDA) has approved a phase I clinical trial to use stem cells to treat crush injury patients with thoracic spinal cord injuries. While a therapy is still a long way off, there is some hope that in the future, spinal cord injury patients will be able to regain most if not all of their previous level of function.

Concept Reinforcement

1. Explain the steps a first responder should take when faced with a spinal cord injury.

2. Explain the steps the physician should take to diagnose a spinal cord injury.

3. Describe the treatment for spinal cord injuries.

Section 3.4 – The Shoulder and Shoulder Injuries

Section Objectives

- Define the general structure of the shoulder joint
- Define several different injuries and treatments for various shoulder joint injuries

Structure of the Shoulder

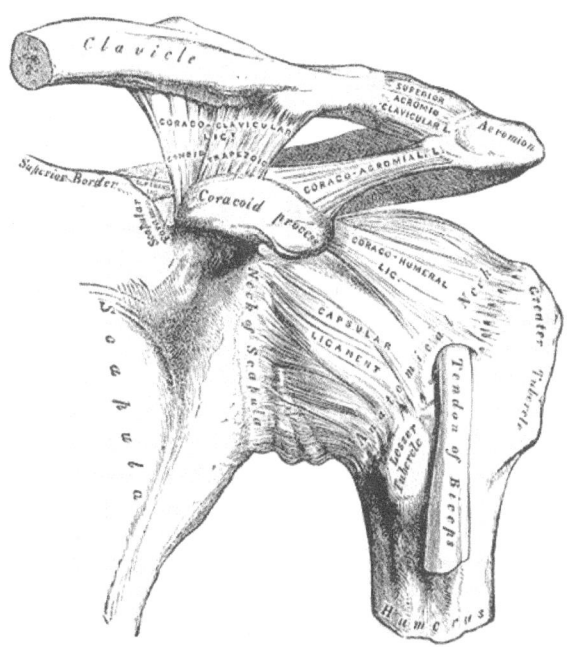

The human shoulder is used for almost every upper body movement. The arms swing from the shoulder to maintain balance while people walk. The shoulder supports the arm when it is raised or while it carries a load. The shoulder is a complex joint where the **scapula**, or shoulder blade, the **clavicle**, or collar bone, and the **humerus**, or upper arm bone, meet. The bones form a **ball and socket** joint which allows the arm to move in three planes. This freedom of movement makes the joint significantly less stable, and it is the most commonly dislocated joint in the body. The joint is surrounded by a number of ligaments to form a capsule, which helps to stabilize the joint.

The bones are stabilized with the muscles and tendons of the **rotator cuff**. The muscles of the rotator cuff are the supraspinatus, subscapularis, infraspinatus, and teres minor. The **supraspinatus muscle** sits atop the ridge of the scapula and attaches to the top of the humerus. The **subscapularis muscle** lies on the **ventral** surface of the scapula, and attaches to the **proximal** ventral surface of the humerus. The **infraspinatus muscle** attaches to the **dorsal** surface of the humerus nearest the top of the humerus and **distal** to the body. The **teres minor muscle** attaches to the distal, dorsal surface of the humerus below the attachment of the infraspinatus. The infraspinatus and teres minor muscles lie on the dorsal surface of the scapula beneath the scapular ridge.

> **Dorsal** indicates the surface closest to the backbone. Its opposite is **ventral**, which means the side closest to the belly.
>
> **Distal** signifies something is far from the centerline of the body. **Proximal** signifies something is close to the center line. For example, the fingers are distal to the body while the shoulder is proximal in comparison.

Injuries and Treatments

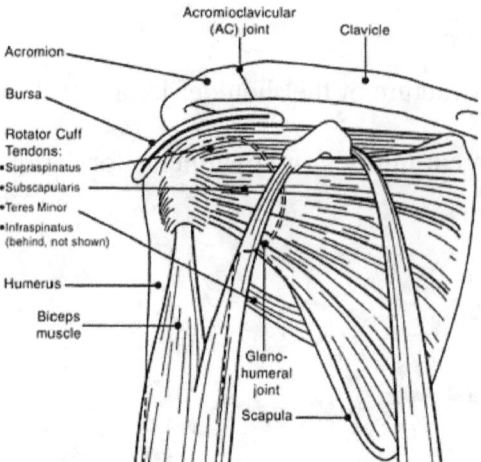

The Shoulder Joint

Impingement syndrome results when a tendon is trapped under the bony acromion, creating pressure or pinching of the tendon.

Impingement syndrome is a fairly common problem of the shoulder joint. Activities that require frequent use of the shoulder, like baseball or tennis, can create muscular imbalances that pull the shoulder joint out of its proper alignment. Age or injury can also cause impingement syndrome. When this occurs, it is possible for a tendon to become trapped beneath the **acromion**, a bony projection from the scapula over the top of the shoulder. The trapped tendon is pinched and becomes inflamed. Movement of the arm or resting the arm in one position for a long time then moving it results in pain.

Joint dislocation is more common at the shoulder than at any other joint. In a dislocation, the head of the humerus separates from the scapula and pops out of the socket. Dislocations are painful, and may result in numbness of the arm and inability to move the arm. In many cases the dislocation is clearly visible. An orthopedic physician will manipulate the arm to put it back in place, a procedure known as **reduction**. The shoulder should be treated with rest, ice, and non-steroidal anti-inflammatory medications (aspirin, acetaminophen, ibuprofen, or naproxen) to reduce swelling and pain.

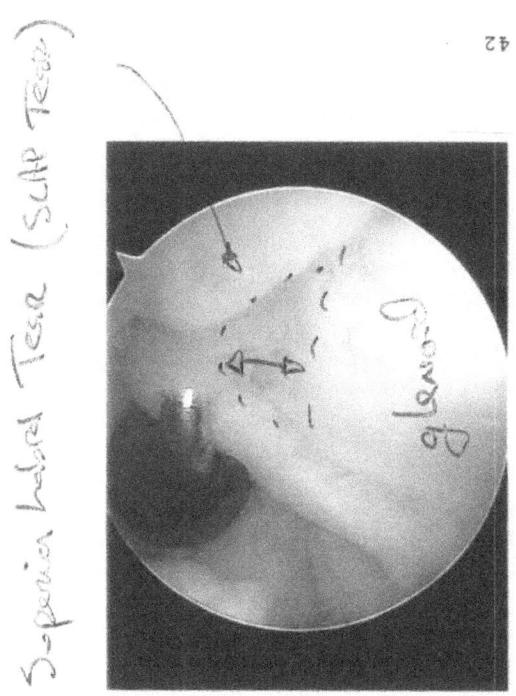

The supraspinatus tendon has been torn free of the humerus.

The small size of the rotator cuff muscles combined with the heavy loads occasionally placed on the shoulder joint makes them subject to injury. Tendon and ligament tears are also fairly common. When the rotator cuff is torn, an orthopedic surgeon will suture the ligaments or tendons back in place. Surgery is followed by an extensive course of regular physical therapy.

Summary

The shoulder is a complex joint where the scapula, or shoulder blade, the clavicle, or collar bone, and the humerus, or upper arm bone, meet to form a ball and socket joint which allows the arm to move in three planes. This freedom of movement makes the joint unstable. The joint is surrounded by a number of ligaments to form a capsule, which helps to stabilize the joint. The bones are stabilized with the muscles and tendons of the rotator cuff: the supraspinatus, subscapularis, infraspinatus, and teres minor. Impingement syndrome occurs when a tendon to become trapped beneath the acromion. The trapped tendon is pinched and becomes inflamed. Movement of the arm or resting the arm in one position for a long time then moving it results in pain. Joint dislocation is more common at the shoulder than at any other joint. In a dislocation, the head of the humerus separates from the scapula and pops out of the socket. An orthopedic physician will perform a reduction. The shoulder should be treated with rest, ice, and non-steroidal anti-inflammatory medication. Tendon and ligament tears are also fairly common. An orthopedic surgeon will suture the ligaments or tendons back in place. Surgery is followed by an extensive course of regular physical therapy.

Concept Reinforcement

1. Describe the bones composing the shoulder and explain how the ball and socket joint is stabilized.

2. Describe the stabilizing muscles of the rotator cuff.

3. Describe the treatment for a dislocated shoulder.

Section 3.5 – The Elbow and Elbow Injuries

Section Objectives

- Describe the structure of the elbow joint

- Explain several different elbow injuries/conditions and their current treatments

Structure of the Elbow

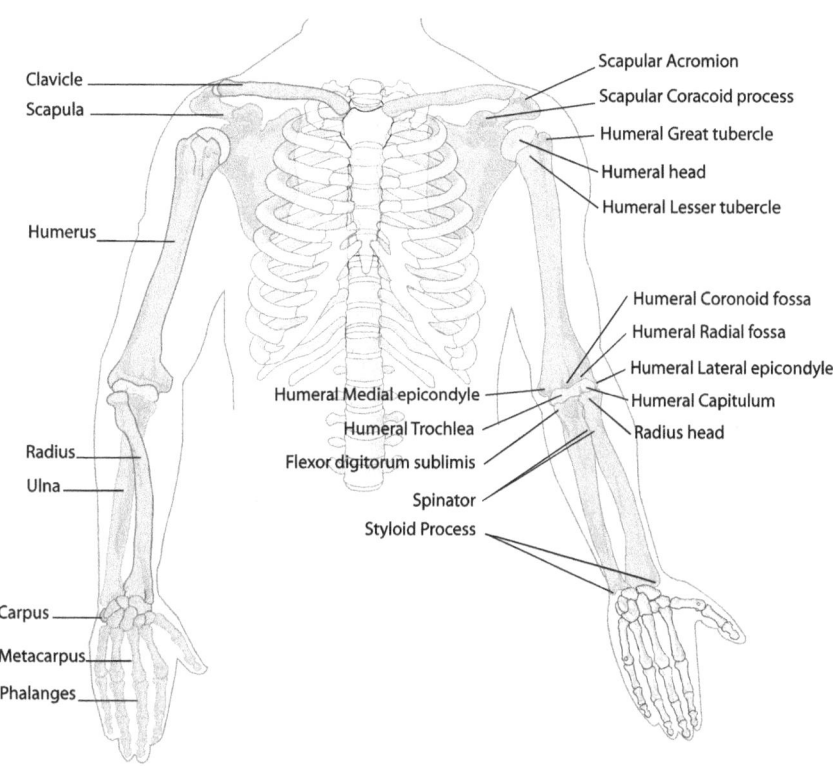

Photograph of Lateral aspect of left human articulation of humerus, radius, and ulna.
Image courtesy of Brian C. Goss.

The elbow is primarily a **hinge joint** between the **humerus**, or upper arm bone, and the **radius** and **ulna**, the two bones of the forearm. The **olecranon** is a bony process that extends from the proximal end of the ulna. It acts in a manner similar to a doorstop, preventing the joint from swinging backwards. When the arm is extended, the olecranon stops against the **olecranon fossa** of the humerus. The elbow is capable of two movements, **flexion and extension**, or bending and straightening, **pronation** and **supination**, a rolling or twisting movement. Pronation and supination are accomplished by the rotation of the radius around the ulna. The elbow is a very stable joint and moves in only one plane. It is stabilized by the **ulnar collateral ligament**, **radial collateral ligament**, and the **annular ligament**.

Injuries of the Elbow

The elbow is the point of origin of the extensor and flexor tendons connecting to the wrist and fingers. These tendons are prone to repetitive motion injuries resulting from participation in sports, especially tennis and golf. **Tennis elbow** is **tendonitis**, inflammation of a tendon, of the flexor tendon. Pain on the inside surface of the forearm at the elbow is the most common symptom. **Golfer's elbow**, on the other hand, is tendonitis of the extensor tendon. Pain in this case is felt along the outer surface of the forearm at the elbow. Rest, ice, compression, elevation, and physical therapy can alleviate both conditions.

Because of the variety of tasks in which the elbow is involved, its location with respect to the body, and the fact that three bones make up the joint, **fractures** are a relatively common injury of the elbow. A fracture can be **simple**, the ends of the broken bone are still in close contact with one another, or **compound**, the broken ends of the bones have separated. Severe compound fractures may include penetration of the skin by the bone. Fractures are serious injuries and should be treated by an orthopedist. An X-ray of the damage will be obtained, and the bones will be properly aligned. The doctor will apply a cast to immobilize the bones to allow them to knit together.

Summary

The elbow is a hinge joint between the humerus, and the radius and ulna. The olecranon extends from the proximal end of the ulna, preventing the joint from swinging backwards. The elbow is capable of flexion and extension, and pronation and supination. The elbow is a very stable joint and moves in only one plane. It is stabilized by the ulnar collateral ligament, radial collateral ligament, and the annular ligament. Tennis elbow and Golfer's elbow are types of tendonitis. Rest, ice, compression, elevation, and physical therapy can alleviate both conditions. Fractures are a relatively common injury of the elbow, and can be simple or compound. An X-ray of the damage will be obtained, the bones will be properly aligned, and the doctor will apply a cast to immobilize the bones to allow them to knit together.

Concept Reinforcement

1. Describe the bones that compose the elbow joint.

2. Describe the ligaments of the elbow.

3. Describe the treatment for tennis elbow.

Section 3.6 – The Body's Core

Section Objectives

- Describe the muscles of the body's core

- Explain how the muscles of the body's core are used to stabilize the body during movement and protect the vital organs beneath

Muscles of the Core

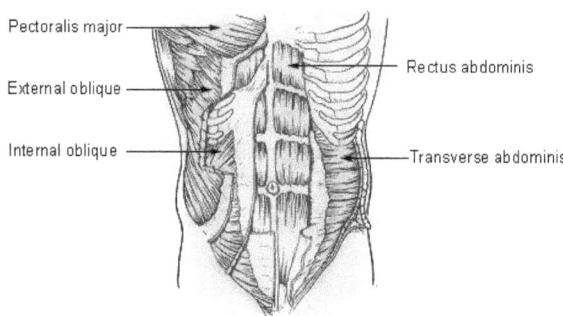

The core muscles of the abdomen include the rectus abdominus, external obliques, internal obliques, and transverse abdominus.

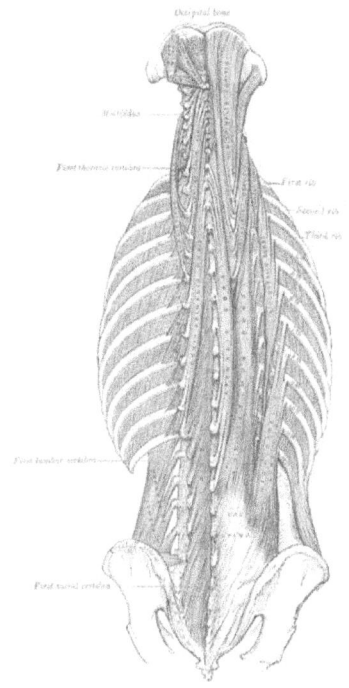

The core muscles of the lower back include the longissimus thoracis, quadrates lumborum, multifidus, and ilio-costalis lumborum. The lower end of the latissimus dorsi (not shown) lies atop the upper portions of the core muscles of the lower back. The latissimus dorsi are not considered part of the core.

The **core** of the body is the region between the pelvis and the ribs. The core muscles of the abdomen include the rectus abdominus, external obliques, internal obliques, and transverse abdominus. The abdominal muscles attach to the ribs and pelvis via short tendons. The rectus abdominus muscles are connected to one another along the midline of the body by a sheet of connective tissue called the **linea alba**, literally the white line. The core muscles of the lower back include the longissimus thoracis, quadrates lumborum, multifidus, and ilio-costalis lumborum. The core muscles of the lower back attach to the ribs and pelvis via short tendons as well. The broad, somewhat triangular sacrospinal tendon anchors the **erector spinae muscles**, the longissimus thoracis, multifidus, and ilio-costalis lumborum to the pelvis.

The spinal column is the sole bony support for the core of the body, so the core is critical in supporting the body in its upright position. The erector spinae muscles are responsible for maintaining the spine in an erect position while standing or sitting. The transverse abdominus muscles of the abdominal muscles are also important to maintaining erect posture by helping to keep the rib cage elevated.

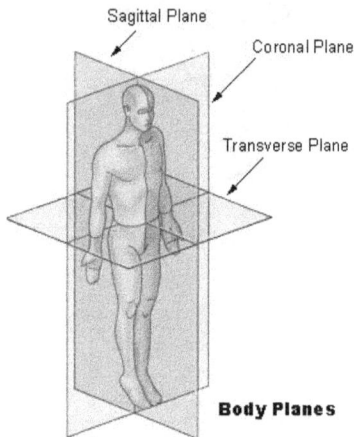

Body Planes

The core permits movement of the body in three planes of movement. The body can bend in the **transverse plane**, forward and backward, the **sagittal plane**, left and right, and the **coronal plane**, twisting while upright. Twisting and bending movements of the body require activation of the core both to create the movement and to stabilize the body through the movement. Sports professionals agree that all sports movements begin with the core and movement of the core in at least one of the three planes. The core stabilizes the body during movement by aligning the hips, spine, and ribs so that the body maintains its balance. It also initiates movements of the extremities by moving the hip to begin leg movements, or transferring power from the hips and legs to the arms for throwing, swinging, or striking motions.

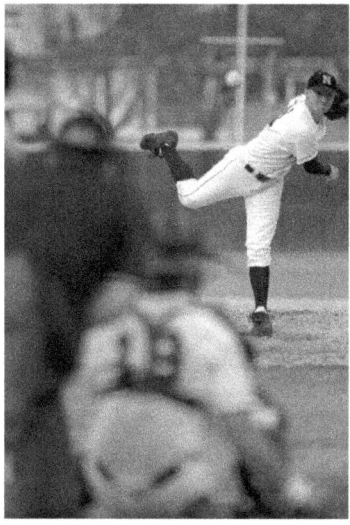

Notice how the hips, spine, and shoulders have rotated through the motion of a pitch. The core both stabilizes the supporting leg and transfers power from the legs and hips to the arms to generate maximum speed and power to throw the ball. The batter will use his core to stabilize his stance and transfer power from the legs to the shoulders and arms to swing the bat.

The muscles of the core provide protection to the **viscera**, the organs of the digestive system. The abdominal organs have no bony protection as do the lungs and heart. Instead, the abdominal muscles must keep the viscera in place, assist them with the movement of food through the intestines and dissipate the force of any impacts to the abdomen. The rectus abdominus, commonly called the "six-pack" muscles, tighten to absorb and dissipate the force of a blow.

Summary

The core of the body is the region between the pelvis and the ribs. The core muscles of the abdomen include the rectus abdominus, external obliques, internal obliques, and transverse abdominus. The rectus abdominus muscles are connected to one another along the midline of the body by a sheet of connective tissue called the linea alba, literally the white line. The core muscles of the lower back include the longissimus thoracis, quadrates lumborum, multifidus, and ilio-costalis lumborum. The broad, somewhat triangular sacrospinal tendon anchors the erector spinae muscles to the pelvis. The core muscles of the abdominals and lower back attach to the ribs and pelvis via short tendons. The spinal column is the sole bony support for the core of the body. The erector spinae and transverse abdominus muscles are responsible for maintaining an erect position while standing or sitting. The core permits movement of the body in three planes of movement. The core stabilizes the body during movement by aligning the hips, spine, and ribs so that the body maintains its balance. It also initiates movements of the extremities by moving the hip to begin leg movements, or transferring power from the hips and legs to the arms for throwing, swinging, or striking motions. The muscles of the core provide protection to the viscera. The abdominal muscles must keep the viscera in place, assist them with the movement of food through the intestines, and dissipate the force of any impacts to the abdomen. The rectus abdominus, commonly called the "six-pack" muscles, tighten to absorb and dissipate the force of a blow.

Concept Reinforcement

1. Describe the muscles of the core.

2. Describe the importance of the core muscles in stability and movement.

3. Describe the protective role of the core.

Section 3.7 – The Wrist

Section Objectives

- Describe the structure of the wrist joint
- Discuss several injuries of the wrist joint and the methods used to treat them

Structure of the Wrist

The wrist is probably the most complex joint in the body. It is capable of a wide range of motions. It is composed of eight bones, the **carpal bones**, arranged in two rows. The **proximal row**, the row nearest the bones of the arm, contains the **scaphoid, lunate**, and **triquetrum** bones. They are connected to the **radius** and **ulna**, the bones of the forearm, by ligaments. There is also a disc of cartilage, the **triangular fibrocartilage complex** between the ulna and the proximal bones of the wrist. The **distal row** of carpal bones, the row closest to the fingers, contains the **trapezium, trapezoid, capitate, hamate**, and **pisiform** bones. They connect to the **metacarpal bones**, the bones of the palm of the hand.

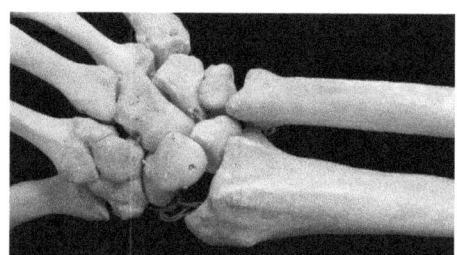

There are 11 ligaments supporting the bones of the wrist. The two most important ligaments are the **ulnar collateral ligament** and the **radial collateral ligament**. The ulnar collateral ligament (UCL) connects the ulna with carpal bones of the outer edge of the wrist, away from the thumb. The radial collateral ligament (RCL) connects the radius with the scaphoid, the carpal bone below the thumb. The UCL also connects to the **transverse carpal ligament**. The transverse carpal ligament is a thick band that runs across the wrist on the palm side. The transverse carpal ligament keeps the tendons responsible for bending the fingers from bowing when the fingers are flexed.

The wrist serves as a passageway for the tendons from the muscles of the forearm that flex and extend the fingers. The **flexor tendons**, the tendons responsible for bending the fingers, pass over the palm side of the wrist and are held in place by the transverse carpal ligament, mentioned above. The **extensor tendons** run over the wrist and the back of the hand to straighten the fingers. The tendons pass through **compartments**, tunnels in the carpal bones that are lined with **tenosynovium**. These are the tunnels of **carpal tunnel syndrome**. Tenosynovium is a slippery substance that reduces friction between the tendons and the carpal tunnels.

The complexity of the wrist joint, combined with the extraordinary amount of use the joint faces over a lifetime makes the wrist especially susceptible to injury. Sprains are common. A **sprain** is an injury to the ligament in which it is stretched beyond its ability to return to its original shape; the ligament undergoes **plastic deformation**. In severe cases the ligaments may actually tear. Sprains are characterized by severe pain, swelling, and loss of function. Sprains are treated using **RICE**; rest, ice, elevation, and compression. Anti-inflammatory medications such as aspirin, acetaminophen, ibuprofen, or naproxen can help reduce the swelling and pain caused by a sprain. Torn ligaments require surgery to repair the ligament followed by a long period of rehabilitation.

Tendonitis is an overuse injury of the tendons. Tendonitis results in pain, inflammation, and swelling of the affected tendon. Tendonitis is treated using RICE and anti-inflammatory medications.

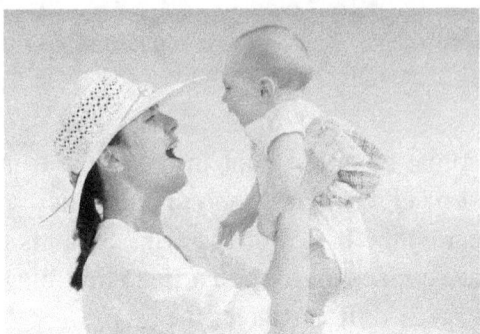

DeQuervain's tenosynovitis is an inflammation of the tenosynovium containing the tendon controlling the thumb. It is common in new mothers because it is caused by overuse of the wrist. The motion of picking up and putting down a baby is especially irritating to this region of the wrist.

DeQuervain's tenosynovitis is an inflammation of the tendons controlling the thumb. It is caused by excessive use of the wrist. New mothers are especially prone to DeQuervain's tenosynovitis because of the motion involved in picking up and putting down a baby. Immobilization of the wrist with or without cortisone injections usually cures the problem. In extreme cases, surgery may be required to provide additional room for the tendon.

Wrist **fractures**, or broken bones, are the most common fractures in the body. The impact of a collision or fall can break one or more of the carpal bones. Pain, swelling, and loss of use of the hand are signs of a wrist fracture. The bones will be set and the hand and lower arm will be immobilized in a cast to allow the bones to heal.

Summary

The wrist is probably the most complex joint in the body. It is capable of a wide range of motions. It is composed of eight carpal bones arranged in two rows. The proximal row consists of the scaphoid, lunate, and triquetrum bones, and the triangular fibrocartilage complex. The distal row of carpal bones consists of the trapezium, trapezoid, capitate, hamate, and pisiform bones. The two most important ligaments of the wrist are the ulnar collateral ligament, which connects the ulna with carpal bones of the outer edge of the wrist, and the radial collateral ligament, which connects the radius with the scaphoid bone below the thumb. The UCL also connects to the transverse carpal ligament, a thick band that runs across the wrist on the palm side that keeps the flexor tendons from bowing when the fingers are flexed. The wrist serves as a passageway for the flexor tendons and the extensor tendons. The tendons pass through compartments lined with tenosynovium.

The complexity of the wrist joint, combined with the extraordinary amount of use the joint faces over a lifetime makes the wrist especially susceptible to injury. Sprains, torn ligaments, tendonitis, DeQuervain's tenosynovitis, and wrist fractures are common. Sprains, tendonitis, and DeQuervain's tenosynovitis are characterized by pain, swelling, and loss of function. They are treated using RICE and anti-inflammatory medications. Torn ligaments require surgery to repair the ligament followed by a long period of rehabilitation. Wrist fractures are set and put in a cast.

Concept Reinforcement

1. Describe the bones that compose the wrist.

2. Describe the ligaments and tendons of the wrist.

3. Describe a sprain and the treatment for a sprain.

Section 3.8 – The Hand

Section Objectives

- Describe the general structure of the hand
- Explain several injuries of the hand and the general treatments used for them

Structure of the Hand

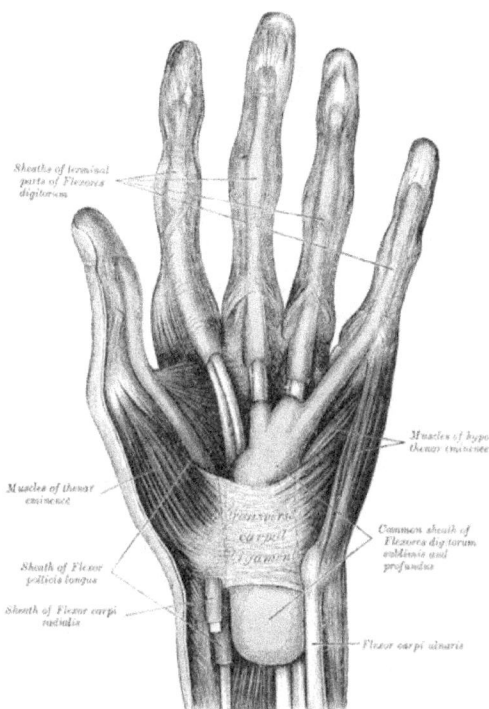

The hand is composed of the metacarpal bones, phalangeal bones, tendons, muscles, and ligaments. It is covered with skin which possesses unique fingerprints, and fingernails.

The hand is probably the most used part of the human body. It is extremely flexible, can grasp and manipulate objects and is used as a sensory device to touch objects. The hand possesses an **opposable thumb**, in other words, it can turn back across the other digits, which greatly increases control over objects gripped in the hand. The hand is made up of the **metacarpal bones**, the bones of the palm of the hand, and the **phalanges**, the bones of the fingers.

The phalanges are stabilized by **collateral ligaments**, ligaments on either side of the joints of the fingers and thumb that prevent lateral movement, and the **volar plate**, a ligament on the palm side of the **proximal interphalangeal joint**. The proximal interphalangeal joint is the first of the two joints on the finger between the first and second phalanges. The volar plate keeps the fingers from bending backwards too far.

The muscles of the hand include the **thenar muscle**, the muscle that controls the thumb, the **hypothenal muscles**, the muscles of the fingers, the **interosseous muscles**, the muscles between the metacarpals, and the **lumbrical muscles**. The fingers are also controlled by the extensor and flexor muscles of the forearm. The flexor and extensor tendons pass through **tenosynovial sheathing**, slippery connective tissue sheaths that reduce friction as the tendons move to control the movements of the fingers.

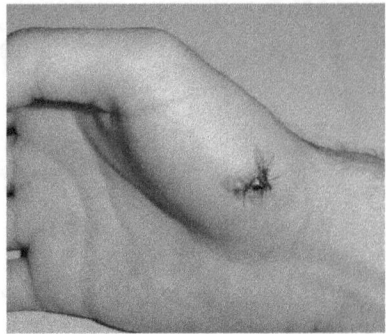

The most common injury to the hand is lacerations.

In a study of hospital emergency rooms, **lacerations**, cuts, are the most common injury to the hand, followed distantly by bruises, fractures, and infections, in that order. Lacerations are cuts, damage to the skin. Bruises are caused by blunt force trauma and are the result of broken blood vessels under the skin. Fractures are broken bones caused by blunt force trauma. Infections are caused by bacteria or viruses introduced to the body when the skin is torn or punctured. The majority of hand injuries are due to blunt force trauma, an impact. Sharp objects cause many of the remaining injuries to the hand.

Broken fingers are fairly common injuries. The phalanges are small bones and are often subjected to large forces. When those forces exceed the ultimate strength of the bone, the bone breaks. Broken fingers are immobilized with a splint and allowed to heal. Metacarpal fractures are also fairly common. In this case, the "hand" is broken. The broken bone in the hand is set and the hand is immobilized in a cast so the bone can heal.

Skier's thumb is caused a torn inner ligament of the thumb. After a tear, the thumb can flex laterally toward the wrist because the stabilization of the ligament is missing. Torn ligaments are treated with surgery and physical therapy.

Tendonitis is an overuse injury and can be seen in athletes, musicians, and others who frequently move their fingers for extended periods of time. Tendonitis is treated with **RICE**; rest, ice, compression, and elevation. Anti-inflammatory medications can help reduce the pain and swelling that accompany tendonitis.

Summary

The hand is probably the most used part of the human body. It is extremely flexible, can grasp and manipulate objects and is used as a sensory device to touch objects. The hand is made up of the metacarpal bones and the phalanges. While some sources include the carpal bones as part of the hand, they have been discussed in a previous section as part of the wrist.

The phalanges are stabilized by collateral ligaments and the volar plate. The muscles of the hand include the thenar muscle, the hypothenal muscles, the interosseous muscles, and the lumbrical muscles. The flexor and extensor tendons pass through tenosynovial sheathing to control the movements of the fingers. Lacerations are the most common injury to the hand, followed distantly by bruises, fractures, and infections, in that order. The majority of hand injuries are due to blunt force trauma, an impact. Sharp objects cause many of the remaining injuries to the hand. Broken fingers are fairly common injuries. Broken fingers are immobilized with a splint and allowed to heal. Metacarpal fractures are also fairly common. In this case, the "hand" is broken. The broken bone in the hand is set and the hand is immobilized in a cast so the bone can heal. Skier's thumb is caused a torn inner ligament of the thumb. After a tear, the thumb can flex laterally toward the wrist. Torn ligaments are treated with surgery and physical therapy. Tendonitis is an overuse injury and can be seen in athletes, musicians, and others who frequently move their fingers for extended periods of time. Tendonitis is treated with RICE, rest, ice, compression, and elevation. Anti-inflammatory medications can help reduce the pain and swelling that accompany tendonitis.

Concept Reinforcement

1. Describe the bones, ligaments, and muscles that compose the hand.

2. Explain the treatment for a broken finger and broken hand.

3. Describe the injuries to the hand in order of prevalence from most to least common.

Section 3.9 – The Spinal Column

Section Objectives

- Discuss the normal curvatures of the spine
- Discuss several common injuries of the spine and how they are currently treated

Shape of the Spine

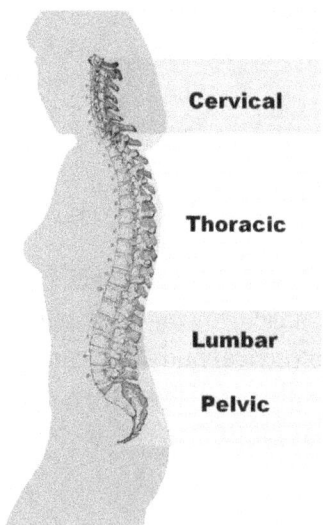

The spine naturally curves backward at the cervical and lumbar vertebrae.

Spinal Curvature

The human spine is not straight, no matter how good the posture of the person. In fact, proper posture allows the spine to curve backwards at the neck and lower back, and slightly forward at the chest and hip level. The curves help to distribute the forces acting on the spine across the entire spinal column rather than at the site at which the force is applied. Direct downward pressure, for example, presses squarely on a cervical vertebra. However, it is directed at an angle onto the next vertebra, reducing its impact. The portion of the force not absorbed by the second vertebra is instead absorbed by the thoracic vertebra in a direct line with the first cervical vertebra. The distribution of the forces continues downward until the entire spine takes up some portion of the load, reducing the stress at the initial site of application. Proper curvature of the spine is important for correct movement of the extremities, proper breathing, and proper digestion. To understand how proper curvature of the spine contributes to movement, breathing, and digestion, it helps to look at examples of improper spinal curvatures and their effects on the body.

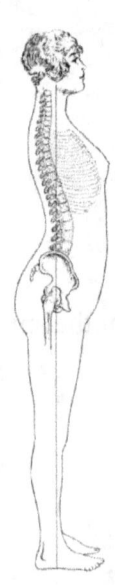

Lordosis

Lordosis, commonly called swayback or saddleback, is an exaggerated inward curvature of the lumbar spine. Lordosis causes lower back pain, and pushes the hips backward. Misalignment of the hips with the vertical body line can make walking and running difficult. Lordosis can usually be treated with exercises to strengthen the abdominal and lower back muscles.

Kyphosis

Kyphosis, or hunchback, is a curvature of the cervical and thoracic vertebrae that rounds the back and lowers the head. Kyphosis causes pain and makes breathing difficult. The rounding of the back and concave compression of the chest make it difficult to completely expand the ribcage, making it difficult to breathe. The ribs press down on the stomach and intestines while the hips often press upward, compressing the **viscera**, the digestive organs, and slowing the passage of food through the digestive tract. Kyphosis can be caused by muscle weakness, causing slouching. It can also be caused by **osteoporosis**, weakening of the bone caused by the loss of calcium, which causes microfractures of the vertebrae. Slouching can be treated with exercises to strengthen the muscles of the upper back.

Scoliosis

Scoliosis is a lateral, or side to side, curvature of the vertebral column. Scoliosis is often a result of birth defects, but can also be caused by injuries, osteoporosis, or abnormal musculature. Depending upon the severity of the curvature, the patient may suffer from pain, uneven hips, shoulders, and/or ribs, or slower neural responses. Uneven hips, shoulders, and ribs can make movement difficult. Breathing and movement of the viscera may be impaired in severe cases. Scoliosis can be treated with a brace while a child or adolescent is growing to try to make the spine curve properly. However, in many cases, surgery is the only treatment.

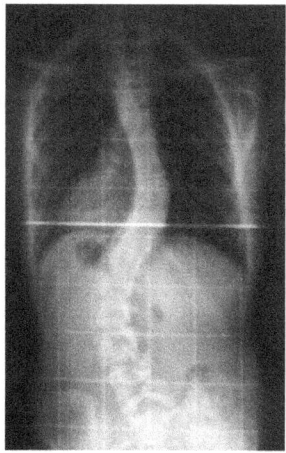

X-ray photograph of a scoliotic spine. Notice the dramatic lateral S-shaped curvature of the spinal column.

Spinal Injuries

Spinal injuries are most commonly caused by vehicular collisions, followed by falls. Injuries of the spine range from the serious to the very serious. Because the spine protects the spinal cord, any injury to the spine can have far-reaching effects. The most common injuries to the spine include: vertebral separation, slipped disc, and fracture of the spine.

Vertebral Separation

Vertebral separation is a dislocation of the vertebrae. Adjoining vertebrae are forced apart to a greater or lesser degree, resulting in an unstable spine. Vertebral separations are relatively rare, and are most common in the **cervical**, or neck, region. The patient is sedated to relax the muscles and the bones are manipulated back into place.

Slipped Disc

The vertebrae are cushioned by **intervertebral discs**, essentially connective tissue sacs containing a gel-like material. Intervertebral discs are found between each vertebra and its neighbor. A **slipped disc** does not really slip. Instead, the disc tears, and the gel-like material inside leaks out and pushes against the spinal cord. Slipped discs are usually caused by improperly lifting heavy or bulky items, especially when turning or twisting. Numbness, weakness, and pain are the most commonly reported symptoms of a slipped disc. If the injury is not severe, ice and hot packs, rest, and over-the-counter anti-inflammatory medications may be all that is required to treat the injury. Physical therapy may be used in more serious injuries. For the most seriously damaged discs, surgical removal of the disc may be required.

Spinal Fracture

A broken back is a very serious injury; in fact, it can be life-threatening. The vertebrae can be cracked, crushed, or have the **spinal processes**, projections from the body of the vertebra to which the muscles of the back are anchored, broken off. Spinal fractures are so serious because they are usually accompanied by spinal cord damage. Spinal fracture treatment is designed around the concern for the spinal cord and potential damage to the cord.

Spinal fractures are treated with immediate immobilization of the head and back with an inflexible cervical collar and backboard. Once at the hospital, the patient should be removed from the backboard as quickly as possible to prevent pain. The doctor should then collect a complete **history** of the injury. In other words, she should ask the patient to describe what happened, any signs or symptoms, and whether there are any sensory or motor deficits. The next step will be to complete a neurological assessment. A **neurological assessment** determines the patient's level of consciousness (alert to unconscious), *mentation* (ability to process thoughts), pupil dilation, motor function (ability to move), sensory responses (responsiveness to soft, sharp, cold, hot, and vibrating objects), and reflex responses (especially to deep tendon reflexes). The level of response will help the doctor gauge whether any accompanying spinal cord injury is incomplete, affecting one side or allowing some level of function, or complete, both sides of the body are unable to move or sense stimuli. She will be able to determine the likely location of the injury based on the areas of the body that are unresponsive. The physical examination is followed by either X-rays or CT scans of the spine. Broken vertebrae may be repaired surgically and fused to nearby vertebrae to stabilize the back and allow for repair to occur. They may be removed surgically and replaced with a bone graft fused to nearby vertebrae. Patients are often placed in **traction**, the application of mechanical force to stretch the spine. Weights are attached to the patient's head and legs to stretch the body. This keeps the vertebrae properly aligned during healing.

Summary

The human spine is curved backwards at the neck and lower back, and slightly forward at the chest and hip level. The curves help to distribute the forces acting on the spine across the entire spinal column rather than at the site at which the force is applied. Proper curvature of the spine is important for correct movement of the extremities, proper breathing, and proper digestion. Lordosis, kyphosis, and scoliosis are abnormal curvatures of the spine that interfere with movement and cause pain. Spinal injuries are most commonly caused by vehicular collisions, followed by falls. Vertebral separation, a dislocation of the vertebrae, is relatively rare, and are most common in the cervical, or neck, region. Slipped discs are usually caused by improperly lifting heavy or bulky items, especially when turning or twisting. A broken back is a very serious injury; in fact, it can be life-threatening. Spinal fractures are so serious because they are usually accompanied by spinal cord damage. Patients are often placed in traction to keep the vertebrae properly aligned during healing.

Concept Reinforcement

1. Explain the importance of the normal curvature of the spine.

2. Describe the differences among lordosis, kyphosis, and scoliosis.

3. Describe a slipped disc and its most likely cause.

Section 3.10 – The Hip

Section Objectives

- Describe the general structure of the hip joint

- Discuss how hip problems can cause dysfunction of other joints in the body and how they are currently treated

Structure of the Hip Joint

The hip is a sturdy ball and socket joint between the **femur**, the upper leg bone, and the **pelvis**, a bony girdle composed of the ischium, ilium, and pubis, attached to the base of the spine. The hip provides support and balance to the body while standing and during locomotion. Unlike the shoulder, the hip joint more completely embeds the femoral head within the socket of the pelvis. This makes the hip joint much more stable than the shoulder. However, the hip is not capable of as wide a range of motion as the shoulder either.

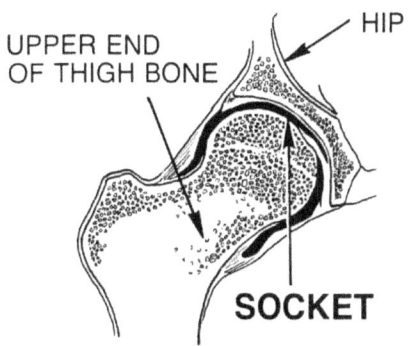

The hip joint is surrounded by a **joint capsule**, which is composed of an outer fibrous connective tissue layer and the inner synovial membrane. The **synovial membrane** secretes **synovial fluid**, a watery fluid that serves as a lubricant between the joints. Synovial fluid also maintains the **articular cartilage** in a hydrated state. The articular cartilage covers the end of the femur and the inner surface of the hip socket.

There are five **ligaments**, tough, relatively inelastic connective tissue, that serve to bind the bones to each other and stabilize the movement of the joint, at the hip joint. The ligaments of the hip are divided into four **extracapsular** ligaments, ligaments outside the joint capsule, and one **intracapsular** ligament, a ligament within the joint capsule.

Common injuries to the hip joint include **stress fractures, osteonecrosis, labral tears**, and **dislocations**. **Hip stress fractures** are overuse injuries, commonly seen in runners. The repetitive pounding of the head of the femur into the socket of the hip causes small cracks to develop. Over time, the joint becomes weakened and may fail. Hip stress fracture is treated with rest and ice, but pain medications should be avoided. This is to make sure painful activities which continue to damage the bone are avoided. **Osteonecrosis** means bone death. Osteonecrosis is caused by a loss of the blood supply to the hip joint. No one knows why this happens. If the blood supply is not repaired, the bone of the joint begins to die, and the joint will fail. Hip osteonecrosis usually requires total hip replacement. The **labrum** is a ring of cartilage around the hip joint that helps to keep the head of the femur in the socket of the hip joint. A **labral tear** can result from weakening due to overuse, as is often the case for runners, or in the event of an acute injury such as a blow or dislocation of the hip. Labral tear is treated with rest, anti-inflammatory medications, and physical therapy. Surgery can be used in severe or unresponsive cases. **Hip dislocations**, a condition in which the head of the femur is forced out of the hip socket, are relatively rare. The hip joint is very strong, and a great deal of force is required to dislocate it. Vehicle collisions and high falls are the most common causes of dislocated hips. Dislocation is treated by manipulating the femoral head back into the socket after anaesthetizing the patient. Physical therapy for two to three months is usually required.

Alterations of the movement of the hips in response to injury alter all of the movements in the body. The repositioning of the hip to avoid pain or to move an injured leg places stress on the muscles of the lower back and causes misalignment of the vertebrae, changes posture, the angle of the shoulders, affecting the movement of the arms. The femur may rotate inward or outward, changing the angle with which the femur meets the tibia and fibula in the knee and placing additional stresses on the knee. The change in the angle of the knee changes the angle with which the tibia and fibula meet the tarsal bones of the ankle. Additional new stresses are placed on the ankle.

Summary

The hip is a sturdy ball and socket joint between the femur, the upper leg bone, and the pelvis, a bony girdle composed of the ischium, ilium, and pubis, attached to the base of the spine. The hip provides support and balance to the body while standing and during locomotion. The hip joint is surrounded by a joint capsule, which is composed of an outer fibrous connective tissue layer and the inner synovial membrane which secretes synovial fluid. Articular cartilage covers the end of the femur and the inner surface of the hip socket. The four extracapsular ligaments and one intracapsular ligament stabilize the movement of the hip. Common injuries to the hip joint include stress fractures, osteonecrosis, labral tears, and dislocations. Hip stress fractures are overuse injuries. Osteonecrosis is caused by a loss of the blood supply to the hip joint. A labral tear can result from weakening due to by overuse or an acute injury. Hip dislocations, relatively rare, are caused by vehicle collisions and high falls. Alterations of the movement of the hips in response to injury alter all of the movements in the body. The repositioning of the hip to avoid pain or to move an injured leg places stress on the muscles of the lower back and causes misalignment of the vertebrae and changes posture, the angle of the shoulders, affecting the movement of the arms.

Concept Reinforcement

1. Describe the bones and ligaments of the hip joint.

2. Explain how hip injuries affect other joints in the body.

3. Describe and explain the treatment for four hip injuries.

Section 3.11 – Structure of the Knee

Section Objectives

- Identify the main structures of the knee joint

Structure of the Knee

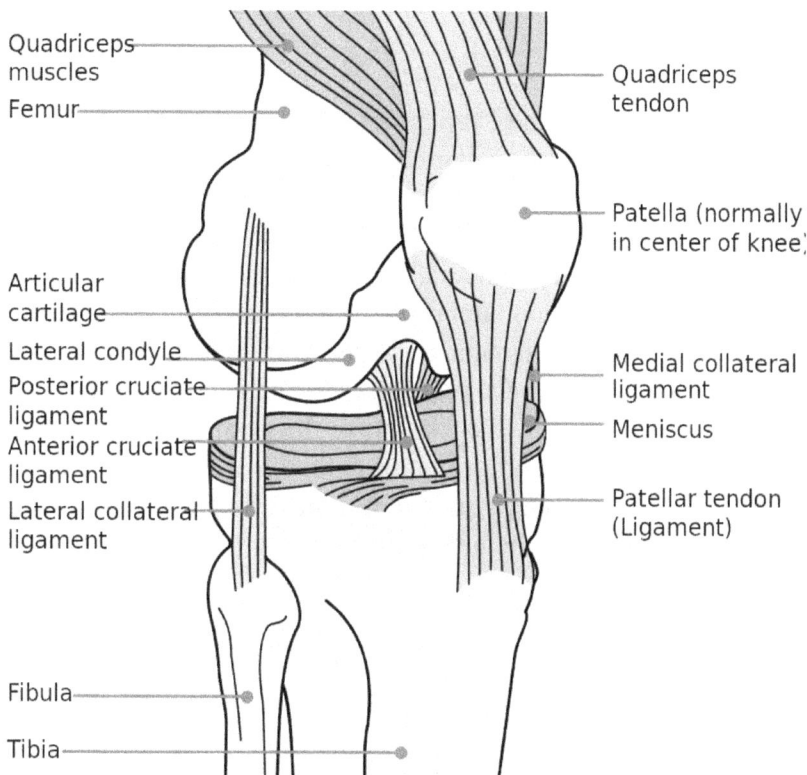

The knee is comprised of four bones, making it one of the most complex joints in the body. The **femur**, or thigh bone, **tibia**, or shin bone, **fibula**, which runs alongside the tibia, and the **patella**, or knee cap, are the bones of the knee. The ends of the femur and tibia are covered with **articular cartilage**, cartilage that cushions the joint and provides a smooth surface over which the joint can glide. There are also two C-shaped rings of cartilage, the **medial meniscus** and the **lateral meniscus**, which fit between the femur and the tibia to help the joint slide more easily. The joint is completely covered by a **bursa**, a thin fluid-filled sac, to help the joint move freely.

The knee is meant to extend forward and flex backward. Four ligaments, two **medial collateral ligaments**, the **anterior cruciate ligament** and **posterior cruciate ligament**, stabilize the joint. The collateral ligaments are found on the inside surface, the medial surface, and the outside surface, the lateral surface, of the knee. They protect against lateral movement of the knee. The anterior cruciate ligament (ACL) anchors the femur to the tibia, attaching the rear of the femur to the forward surface of the tibia. The ACL prevents the femur from sliding forward on the tibia. The posterior cruciate ligament (PCL) anchors the forward edge of the femur to the rear of the tibia. The PCL prevents the femur from sliding backward on the tibia.

The patella is held in place by the tendons of the four heads of the **quadriceps muscle**, or thigh muscle, and the **patellar tendon**, the tendon that attaches the patella to the tibia. The patella acts as a fulcrum to increase the leverage that the quadriceps muscle can apply to the tibia. The quadriceps and the **hamstrings**, the muscles of the back of the thigh, help hold the knee in place. The hamstrings are responsible for flexing the knee.

Summary

The knee is comprised of four bones, the femur, tibia, fibula, and patella. The ends of the femur and tibia are covered with articular cartilage. There are also two C-shaped rings of cartilage, the medial meniscus and the lateral meniscus, which fit between the femur and the tibia to help the joint slide more easily. The joint is completely covered by a bursa. The knee is stabilized by two medial collateral ligaments, the anterior cruciate ligament and posterior cruciate ligament. The collateral ligaments protect against lateral movement of the knee. The anterior cruciate ligament prevents the femur from sliding forward on the tibia. The posterior cruciate ligament prevents the femur from sliding backward on the tibia. The patella is held in place by the tendons of the quadriceps muscle, and the patellar tendon. The patella acts as a fulcrum to increase the leverage that the quadriceps muscle can apply to the tibia. The quadriceps and the hamstrings help hold the knee in place. The quadriceps extend the knee while the hamstrings flex the knee.

Concept Reinforcement

1. Describe the bones of the knee joint.

2. Describe the ligaments of the knee joint and their functions.

3. Describe the muscles and tendons of the knee joint and their functions.

Section 3.12 – Knee Injuries

Section Objectives

- Explain several common injuries to the knee joint and treatments

Knee Injuries

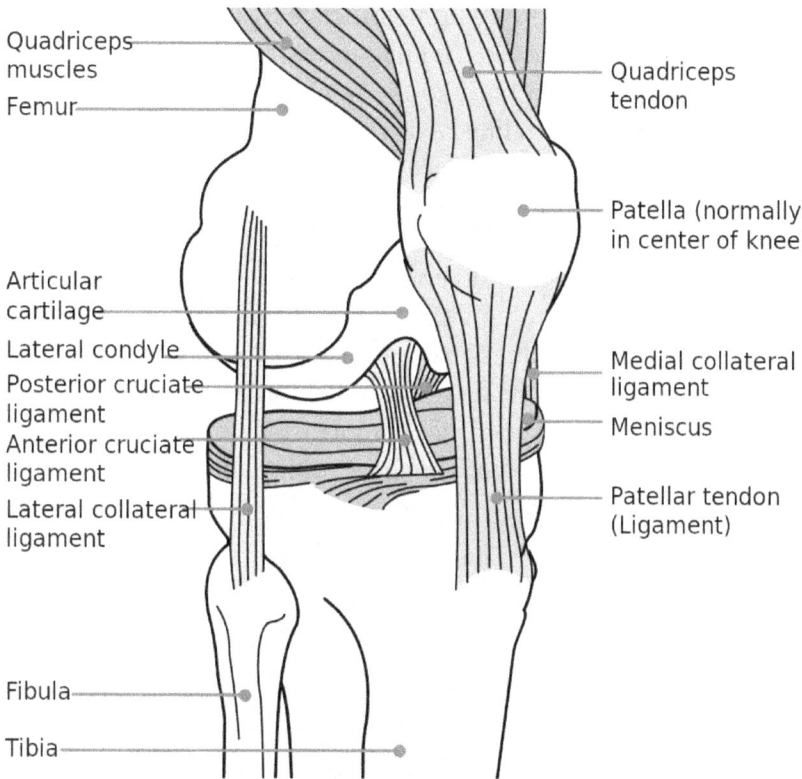

The complexity of the knee coupled with its near constant use result in it being one of the most commonly injured joints in the body. In most cases, the injury results from a blow to the knee. In the following discussion, we will examine several common knee injuries and their treatments.

Osteoarthritis, the wearing away of the cartilage, is the most common knee problem. Knee cartilage wears away due to overuse or injuries. Excessive weight gain can cause overuse injury to the knee resulting in osteoarthritis. The bones begin to rub against one another directly, without the friction- and impact-reducing benefit of the articular cartilage. Over-the-counter anti-inflammatory medications and pain relievers can be used to reduce the pain and swelling that accompanies osteoarthritis. Weight loss can reduce the severity of osteoarthritis. Exercises that improve the strength of the muscles around the knee can improve joint stability and reduce friction. Knee replacement surgery is becoming common in severe cases of osteoarthritis.

Chondromalacia, a softening of the cartilage, is usually caused by injury, overuse, or muscle weakness. It is not uncommon for a portion of the **meniscus**, the C-shaped pieces of cartilage between the femur and the tibia, to be torn when the leg twists under a load. The resulting chondromalacia can be treated with exercises to strengthen the muscles while allowing the cartilage to heal itself. In severe cases, surgery may be required to repair the cartilage.

Ligament injuries are **sprains**, small tears or stretching of the ligament, or more severe tears. The ligaments of the knee are frequently injured in sports such as football and hockey, and automotive collisions. Anterior cruciate ligament (ACL) sprains and tears are usually caused by a twisting motion. Posterior cruciate ligament sprains (PCL) and tears are caused by a blow to the leg that forces the knee forward. Sprains and tears of the collateral ligaments are usually caused by a blow to the outside of the knee. Ligament injuries are treated with ice to reduce the swelling. A brace and exercise therapies to strengthen the muscles help stabilize the knee and reduce the strain on the ligaments. In severe cases, surgery is required to repair the ligaments.

Tendons are occasionally injured in the knee, typically by overuse. **Tendonitis**, inflammation of the tendon, is a relatively common sports injury that causes pain and swelling. The result is a weakened tendon. Tendons that are overused and weakened are susceptible to stretching or tearing. In older people, tendons can be torn while trying to land during a fall. Tendonitis is treated with **RICE**, rest, ice, compression, and elevation. Over-the-counter anti-inflammatory medications help reduce the swelling. In the case of a ruptured tendon, surgery will be required.

Summary

The complexity of the knee coupled with its near constant use result in it being one of the most commonly injured joins in the body. In most cases, the injury results from a blow to the knee. Osteoarthritis, the most common knee problem occurs when knee cartilage wears away due to overuse or injuries. It is treated with over-the-counter anti-inflammatory medications and pain relievers, weight loss, exercise, and knee replacement surgery. Chondromalacia is usually caused by injury, overuse, or muscle weakness. Chondromalacia can be treated with exercises or surgery. Ligament injuries, sprains or more severe tears, are treated with ice, a brace, and exercise therapies. In severe cases, surgery is required to repair the ligaments. Tendons are typically injured by overuse. Tendonitis causes pain and swelling. Tendonitis is treated with RICE, over-the-counter anti-inflammatory medications, or in severe cases with surgery.

Concept Reinforcement

1. Describe osteoarthritis of the knee and its treatment.

2. Describe knee ligament injuries and their treatment.

3. Describe knee tendon injuries and their treatment.

Section 3.13 – The Ankle and Ankle Injuries

Section Objectives

- Explain the general anatomical make-up of the ankle joint
- Discuss several different injuries and conditions associated with the ankle joint and current treatments

Anatomy of the Ankle

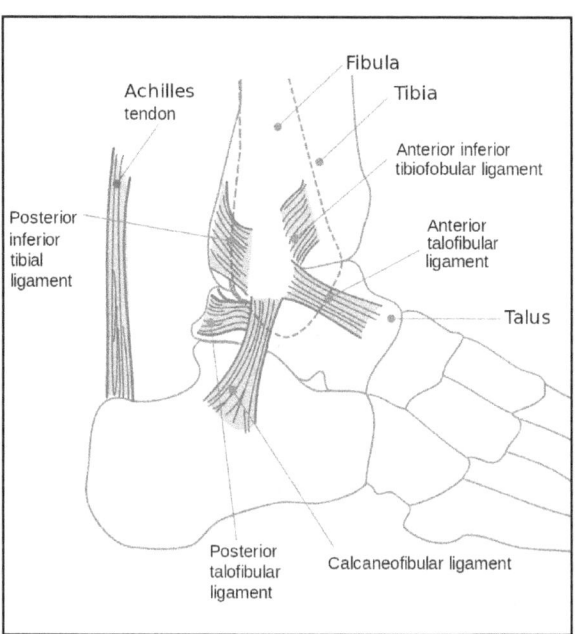

The ankle is really made up of two joints, the **subtalar joint**, and the **true ankle joint**. The true ankle joint includes the tibia and fibula of the lower leg with the **talus**. The true ankle joint permits flexion and extension of the foot. The subtalar joint includes the talus and the **calcaneus**. The calcaneus is found directly beneath the talus, and forms the backward projection of the heel of the foot. The subtalar joint is responsible for the ability of the foot to move from side to side.

The ankle is stabilized by several ligaments. The anterior and posterior tibiofibular ligaments bind the tibia and fibula to one another. The anterior and posterior talofibular ligaments, and calcenofibular ligament, provide lateral stability to the ankle. The deltoid ligament (not shown in the figure) binds the inside surface of the fibula to the inside surface of the talus to prevent the ankle from rolling inward.

The **Achilles tendon** attaches the **gastrocnemius**, **soleus**, and **plantaris** muscles, the muscles of the calf, to the calcenous at the heel. The Achilles tendon is the thickest and strongest tendon in the body. The Achilles tendon is responsible for flexing, or pointing, the foot.

Ankle Injuries

Ankle injuries include injuries to the bones, ligaments, and tendons of the ankle. The bones of the ankle may be broken, usually as the result of a blow, although occasionally as a result of extreme flexing of the ankle. Martial arts practitioners occasionally break the calcaneus when performing a back roundhouse kick. While a broken ankle is extremely painful, it is not uncommon for the patient to be capable of walking on it. However, walking on a broken ankle will only worsen the injury. A broken ankle should have the bones aligned properly by a physician, followed by immobilization in a cast until the bones can heal.

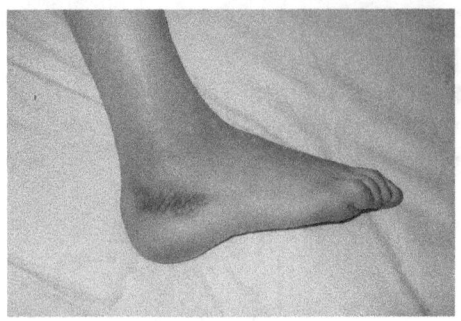

Ligament injuries include sprains and tears. Ankle sprains are common. When the ankle is rolled over laterally, the talofibular ligaments can be stretched or torn, resulting in a sprained ankle. The severity of the sprain is graded as Level 1, 2, or 3. A Level 1 or 2 sprain results when the ligaments are stretched, but not torn. These sprains usually heal fairly quickly and completely. Rest, ice, compression, and elevation, **RICE**, is the preferred method of treatment. A Level 3 sprain results when the ligament is torn. Level 3 sprains take much longer to heal, and in severe cases may require surgery. Sprains are extremely painful and the patient cannot place any weight on the injured foot or walk.

Tendon injuries of the ankle include tendonitis and tendon ruptures. Tendonitis is an overuse injury. The tendon becomes inflamed, with swelling, heat, and pain in the area. Tendonitis is treated with RICE and over-the-counter anti-inflammatory drugs. Inflamed tendons become weakened, and if the overuse is not corrected, the tendon can rupture. Rupture of the Achilles tendon is especially traumatic. The Achilles tendon is critical in walking and running. When the tendon ruptures, it must be repaired surgically.

Summary

The ankle is composed of two joints, the subtalar joint, responsible for the ability of the foot to move from side to side, and the true ankle joint, which permits flexion and extension of the foot. The true ankle joint includes the tibia and fibula of the lower leg with the talus. The subtalar joint includes the talus and the calcaneus. The calcaneus forms the backward projection of the heel of the foot. The anterior and posterior talofibular ligaments, deltoid ligament, and calcenofibular ligament provide stability to the ankle. The Achilles tendon, the thickest and strongest tendon in the body, attaches the muscles of the calf to the calcenous. Ankle injuries include a broken ankle, sprains and tears, and tendonitis. Broken ankles, sprains, and tears are immobilized. Tendonitis is treated with RICE, over-the-counter anti-inflammatory medication, and surgery in severe cases.

Concept Reinforcement

1. Describe the two joints of the ankle and the bones of each joint.

2. Describe the ligaments of the ankle and their functions.

3. Explain the difference between a broken ankle and a sprain.

Section 3.14 – The Foot and Foot Injuries

Section Objectives

- Describe the structure of the foot and discuss how it is susceptible to injury
- Discuss common foot conditions and injuries and their treatments

Anatomy of the Foot

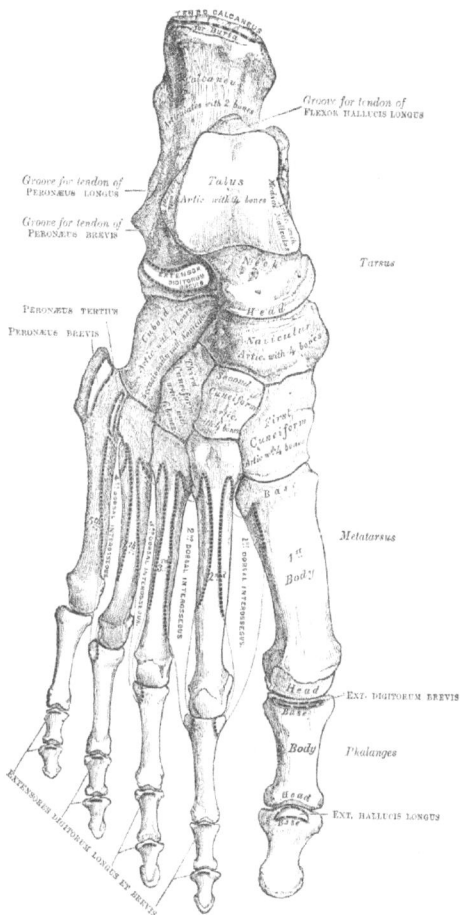

The foot is a complex structure composed of a large number of bones. The bones of the feet include five tarsal bones, five metatarsal bones, and five phalanges. The five tarsal bones are the **navicular bone**, the **cuboidal bone**, and the **first, second, and third cuneiform bones**. The navicular and cuboidal bones abut the two tarsal bones of the ankle, the talus and the calcaneus. The **first metatarsus** is the metatarsal connected to the **phalanges** of the big toe. It is the primary weight-bearing bone of the foot, and commensurately thick and heavy. It plays the greatest role in propulsion, and is the site of attachment for several tendons. The other metatarsals provide increased stability to the foot to keep it from rolling over on its side during locomotion. The phalanges are the bones of the toes.

Many small ligaments hold the bones of the foot in place. Most of them make up part of the joint capsule which surrounds and lubricates each joint. There are many tendons in the foot as well. Some of the tendons attach muscles found within the foot to the bones of the foot. These muscles and tendons are called **intrinsic muscles** and **intrinsic tendons**, because they are intrinsic to, or part of, the foot. Tendons also reach the foot from muscles of the lower leg, especially the calf muscles. These tendons and muscles are referred to as **extrinsic muscles** and **tendons**, because they arise outside the foot itself. The most important extrinsic tendon is the Achilles tendon which attaches the muscles of the calf to the calcaneus. The **plantar fascia** is a tendon that runs along the bottom of the foot, and is originally part of the Achilles tendon during childhood. As people age, the plantar fascia becomes independent from the Achilles tendon.

Foot Injuries

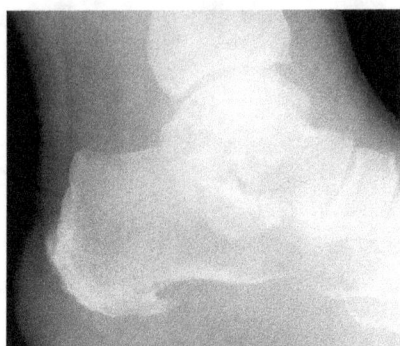

The X-ray above shows a heel spur on the lower surface of the calcaneus. Heel spurs such as this one are commonly seen in patients suffering from plantar fasciitis.

Foot injuries can occur in the forefoot, midfoot, or hindfoot. Injuries to the foot include:

- Turftoe – a sprain of the metatarsal/phalangeal joint at the base of the big toe. It is caused when the toe is bent too far upward. Treatment includes rest, ice, compression, and elevation, **RICE**. Compression is usually accomplished by taping the toe and forefoot. The injury is called turftoe because it was common in athletes playing on artificial turf.

- Blisters – a burn usually caused by friction that results in fluid buildup under the skin. Small blisters can be allowed to heal on their own. Larger blisters are treated by breaking the blister and allowing it to drain, application of antiseptic, and bandaging.

- Stress fractures – small cracks in the bones of the foot resulting from overuse and/or insufficient calcium and vitamin D in the diet. Stress fractures are treated with rest to allow the cracks to heal.

- Heel spurs – an overuse injury in which a bony outgrowth occurs where a chronically inflamed tendon or ligament attaches to the bone. Heel spurs can be quite painful. Treatment for heel spurs includes taping the injured area to reduce use, anti-inflammatory medication, and physical therapy. When these fail, the heel spur is removed surgically.

- Plantar fasciitis – an overuse injury common in runners. The planter fascia becomes inflamed, causing pain, especially first thing in the morning and after long rest periods. Plantar fasciitis is treated with anti-inflammatory medication, stretching exercises, and foot strengthening exercises. Using shoes with adequate cushioning while running or if a job requires long periods of standing and walking help prevent plantar fasciitis.

Summary

The foot is a complex structure composed of a large number of bones. The bones of the feet include five tarsal bones, navicular bone, the cuboidal bone, and the first, second, and third cuneiform bones, five metatarsal bones, and five phalanges. The first metatarsus is connected to the phalanges of the big toe, and is the primary weight-bearing bone of the foot. Many small ligaments hold the bones of the foot in place. Most of them make up part of the joint capsule which surrounds and lubricates each joint. The many tendons in the foot are classified as intrinsic or extrinsic tendons. The most important extrinsic tendon is the Achilles tendon which attaches the muscles of the calf to the calcaneus. The plantar fascia is a tendon that runs along the bottom of the foot, and is originally part of the Achilles tendon during childhood. As people age, the plantar fascia becomes independent from the Achilles tendon. Foot injuries include turftoe, blisters, stress fractures, heel spurs, and plantar fasciitis. Overuse injuries and sprains like turftoe, heel spurs, stress fractures, and plantar fasciitis are treated with rest, compression, and anti-inflammatory medications. Blisters may be allowed to heal on their own, or they may be drained and treated with antiseptic to prevent infection.

Concept Reinforcement

1. Describe the bones of the foot.

2. Describe the cause and treatment of heel spurs.

3. Explain the difference between an intrinsic and an extrinsic muscle or tendon.

Section 3.15 – Osteoarthritis

Section Objectives

- Describe the mechanism behind osteoarthritis related to sports injuries

Osteoarthritis

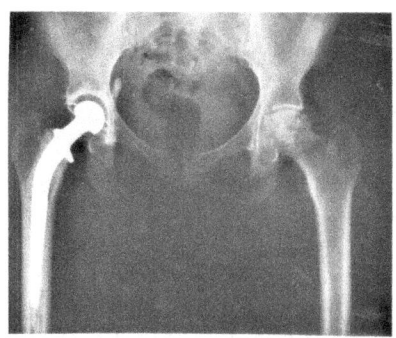

Total hip joint replacement. The patient's right hip (on the left in the photograph) has been replaced, with the "ball" of this ball-and-socket joint replaced by a metal head that is set in the thighbone or femur and the socket replaced by a white plastic cup. Although not the case here, the hip prosthetic can also be made of ceramic which rarely wears out during the patient's lifetime. During the operation, a bonding cement is used to fix the cup to the patient's remaining hip bone. One of the leading reasons for hip replacement is osteoarthritis of the hip joint in which virtually all of the cartilage around the top of the femur bone deteriorates over time, leaving a grinding bone-on-bone situation with the top surface of the femur ball usually taking on an appearance similar to sandpaper. This can result in a narrowing of the space in the hip's natural ball-and-socket joint structure, thereby causing limited mobility of the hip and an intense amount of constant pain in the hip joint.

Osteoarthritis is a condition in which the articular cartilage of the joint on the end of the bone has been worn away by disease, overuse, or injury. The result is that the bones grind on one another rather than gliding smoothly past one another when the joint is used. Over time, the bone looks like used sandpaper. Movement is painful, and often the range of motion of the joint becomes limited. The body's immune system may act to remove some of the damaged tissue, causing additional inflammation and pain. As the body attempts to regrow lost tissue, bone spurs may develop. Bone spurs can cause even more pain, further reduce mobility of the joint, and are prone to breaking. If a bone spur breaks off, the bony fragments may become lodged in the joint. They may grind against the bones of the joint, damage the ligaments and tendons, or cause the joint to lock. Because movement can be so painful, patients frequently reduce movement of the affected joints. The reduced movement leads to weakening of the ligaments, and **atrophy**, or decrease in size and strength, of the nearby muscles.

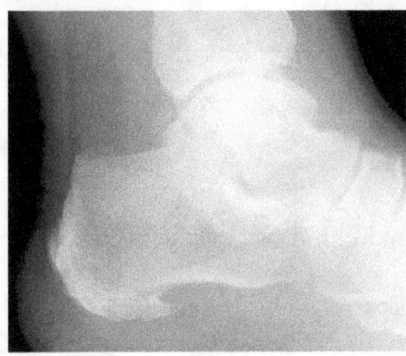

Heel spurs are bony growths caused by the body's attempt to heal bone damage.

Osteoarthritis and Sports Injuries

Sports injuries can lead to the development of osteoarthritis in later life. Osteoarthritis is common in running and football. Running, especially long distance running, causes overuse injuries to the ankles, knees, hips, and lower spine. The constant jarring impact of the foot hitting the ground compresses the joints, weakens the ligaments, and damages the cartilage. Weakened ligaments destabilize the joint and permit contact between the ends of the bones. Over time, the articular cartilage of the joint is worn down, and the bones can begin to grind on one another directly. The result is osteoarthritis.

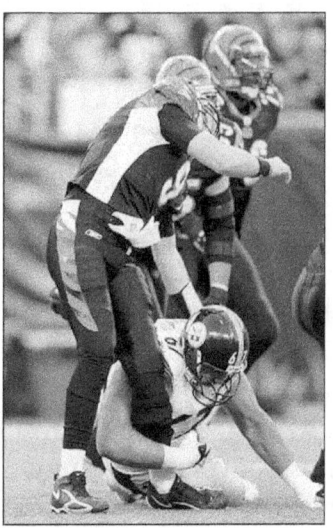

Carson Palmer of the Cincinnati Bengals tore his anterior cruciate ligament, medial collateral ligament, and cartilage in the knee, as well as dislocating his patella, during a game against the Pittsburgh Steelers in 2006. Injuries of this type can lead to osteoarthritis in later life.

Football injuries tend to cause osteoarthritis to develop in a slightly different way. Football injuries tend to be **traumatic**, the result of a blow. Some of these injuries directly damage the cartilage, causing tears or completely separating the cartilage from the bone. Other injuries cause ligament damage. One of the more common ligament injuries in football is a torn anterior cruciate ligament. The tear destabilizes the joint, and allows the articular cartilage of the femur to rub against the articular cartilage of the tibia. Over time, the articular cartilage can wear away, resulting in osteoarthritis.

Osteoarthritis Treatment

Osteoarthritis affects over 27 million people in the US and accounts for approximately one quarter of doctor's office visits. Health professionals estimate that 80% of the US population will have osteoarthritis by the time they reach age 65, although only 48% of the population will actually report symptoms. The number of hospital stays resulting from osteoarthritis has more than doubled from 1993 to 2006.

Treatment for osteoarthritis typically begins with **non-steroidal anti-inflammatory drugs** (NSAIDS), aspirin, acetaminophen, ibuprofen, or naproxen. They can reduce the immune response, reduce the inflammation, and alleviate the pain of osteoarthritis in most cases. When NSAIDS are not enough, doctors may resort to using **corticosteroids**, steroid anti-inflammatory medications that mimic the effects of steroids produced naturally by the adrenal gland. The benefits of steroids for osteoarthritis treatment are controversial, and the risks probably outweigh the benefits, but the decision should be made by the patient and the doctor based on the individual circumstances of the case. Joint replacement surgery is the last resort for treatment of osteoarthritis. Hips, knees, and shoulders can be replaced with artificial joints. The availability of joint replacement surgery and its increasing success is the reason for the more than doubling of the number of hospital stays related to osteoarthritis.

Summary

Osteoarthritis is a condition in which the articular cartilage of the joint on the end of the bone has been worn away by disease, overuse, or injury. Movement is painful, and often the range of motion of the joint becomes limited. The body's immune system may act to remove some of the damaged tissue, causing additional inflammation and pain. As the body attempts to regrow lost tissue, bone spurs may develop. Because movement can be so painful, reduced movement leads to weakening of the ligaments, and atrophy of the nearby muscles. Osteoarthritis is common in running and football. Running causes overuse injuries to the ankles, knees, hips, and lower spine. It weakens the ligaments, and damages the cartilage. Over time, the articular cartilage of the joint is worn down, resulting in osteoarthritis. Football injuries tend to be traumatic, directly damaging the cartilage or ligaments. Ligament damage destabilizes the joint, and allows the articular cartilage of the bones to rub against one another, resulting in osteoarthritis. Osteoarthritis affects over 27 million people in the US, accounts for approximately one quarter of doctor's office visits, and will affect 80% of the US population. Treatment for osteoarthritis typically begins with NSAIDS to reduce the immune response, reduce the inflammation, and alleviate the pain. When NSAIDS are not enough, doctors may resort to using corticosteroids, but the benefits of steroids for osteoarthritis treatment are controversial. Joint replacement surgery is the last resort for treatment of osteoarthritis. Hips, knees, and shoulders can be replaced with artificial joints. The availability of joint replacement surgery and its increasing success is the reason for the more than doubling of the number of hospital stays related to osteoarthritis.

Concept Reinforcement

1. Describe osteoarthritis.

2. Describe the treatment of osteoarthritis.

3. Explain how sports injuries can result in osteoarthritis.

Appendix

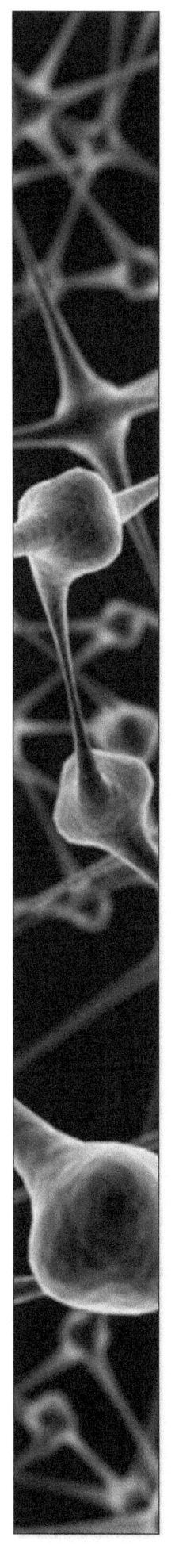

Introduction to Sports Medicine Answer Key – Unit 1

Section 1.1

1. Any of the following: Athletic Training, Biomechanics, Chiropractics, Ergonomics, Exercise Physiology, Kinesiology, Massage Therapy, Occupational Therapy, Orthopedics, Personal Training, Sports Physician, Physical Therapy, Teaching, Coaching, Sports Psychology

2. To treat the athletes competing in the 1928 St. Moritz winter Olympics

3. The medical advances made by sports medicine practitioners can be used on everyone, whether or not they are athletes.

Section 1.2

1. Leadership, training, strategy, counselor, organizer, enforcer of rules

2. Massage therapists help athletes with flexibility and avoid injury by working out knots in the muscles and increasing blood flow.

3. Bachelor's degree in athletic training, physical education, education science, or health. A certified athletic trainer must pass the NATABOC certification exam.

4. Kinesiology is the study of movement. Kinesiologists work with athletes to ensure proper movement and decrease the risk of injury. They also use their knowledge of movement to develop new training techniques and design new equipment.

Section 1.3

1. The joints allow us to move.

2. This theory describes the relationship between the joints of the body and how a problem in one joint can affect other joints.

3. If a joint is not moving the way it is supposed to, the body adapts by forcing the next joint to absorb the stress of the movement. This can cause pain in the joint that is absorbing the stress, especially if it is not designed to move that way.

4. Repetitive action, trauma, crystal deposits in the tissues, friction in the joint, systemic diseases.

Section 1.4

1. The process of helping a person recover full function after an injury.

2. She observed that muscles must be allowed to heal completely before beginning a strengthening program.

3. The fourth rehabilitation theory includes what she learned about the muscles and joints, as well as how the brain controls movement.

Section 1.5

1. Range of motion is the ability of a joint to move and is an isolated measure of movement that can occur at a joint.

2. Saggital, Frontal (coronal), Transverse

3. Flexibility is the ability of the joint to move. The muscles and tissues surrounding the joint must be able to stretch and contract to allow movement of the joint. If the muscles and tendons are not flexible, the mobility of the joint will be limited.

Section 1.6

1. Muscle force capability is the ability of the muscle to generate force. This capability is limited by muscles that are too short or too long. Maximum muscle force capability occurs when the thin and thick muscle fibers overlap as much as they are able to, forming bridges.

2. An electric circuit that provides a path for electrons to return to the source of power. There is no break in the circuit so electrons will flow.

3. Thixotropy is loss of flexibility resulting from a muscle being immobilized for a long period of time. Hypertrophy is the overdevelopment of muscle.

Section 1.7

1. The number of times your heart beats in a minute.

2. Resting heart rate: heart rate when completely at rest.
   Maximum heart rate: the fastest the heart can beat.
   Training (or target) heart rate: the heart rate for various types of training.

3. The RPE scale is a measure of exertion based on the perception of the athlete.

Section 1.8

1. Body mass index is a measure of an individual's body mass in weight and in relationship to their stature (height).

2. Any three of the following:
   Height-Weight: moderately accurate.
   Waist-hip ratio: moderately accurate.
   Pinch Test: not very accurate.
   Bioelectrical impedance test: not very accurate
   Immersion test: highly accurate
   Bod Pod: highly accurate

3. Many BMI measures to not take into account the mass of an individual that has more bone or muscle weight than fat weight. The exceptions are the immersion test and bod pod.

Section 1.9

1. Atomic, molecular, cellular, tissue/system, whole body

2. Cells that are similar to one another in appearance, function and embryonic origin group together to form tissues.

3. The whole body is easily observed and measured. The measurements taken at the whole body level indicate what is happening at the other four levels in the body. The sports medicine professional can use that information to modify nutrition and workout programs.

Section 1.10

1. Power is a measure of the ability to move a sub-maximal load.

2. Speed is a measure of how quickly a person can sprint from point A to point B in a straight line. Agility is the ability to quickly change direction while sprinting.

3. Power: Vertical jump test.
   Speed: 40 yard sprint time for football players.
   Agility: Pro Agility Drill.

Section 1.11

1. The FMS is a method for screening the way a patient moves.

2. Functional Movement
   Functional Performance
   Functional Skills

3. Deep squat, Inline lunge, Shoulder mobility, Hurdle step, Rotary stability, Trunk stability pushup, Active straight leg raise.

Section 1.12

1. To increase tissue temperature, increase muscle extensibility (ability to stretch), prepare the body to move in a single-leg stance, and prepare the central nervous system for higher levels of activity

2. Active, Static, Passive, Dynamic

3. Passive-static stretching requires another person or a stretching tool to provide the force required for the stretch. Passive dynamic stretching requires you to provide your own force.

Section 1.13

1. To correct faulty movement resulting from an injury to a joint.

2. The assessment provides the information the therapist needs to design the corrective exercise program.

3. The exercises from the corrective exercise program are designed to strengthen the injured joint. They continue to help strengthen the joint and prevent further injury even after rehabilitation is complete.

Section 1.14

1. Each muscle fiber contains numerous actin and myosin filaments, special proteins that can form crosslinks. When the two filaments form crosslinks, the heads on the myosin filaments bend, sliding the two filaments past one another. The heads detach, reposition themselves, and begin the process again. This ratchet- like sliding movement is how muscles contract.

2. Age, adiposity, and exercise

3. Fatty deposits within and between the muscle fibers increase or maintain the cross-sectional area of the muscle without contributing to strength.

4. Such training increases the cross- sectional area of type II fibers in the muscle, increases the number of muscle fibers activated during a movement, and increases myofibrillar packing, the number of actin and myosin filaments packed into a muscle cell. More actin and myosin filaments means more crossbridges that can be formed, increasing muscular strength.

Section 1.15

1. RDA is the recommended daily allowance of various nutrients, including vitamins and minerals.

2. Athletes use more energy than the average person, therefore require more nutrients to provide energy to the body. The RDA is based on the nutritional needs of a person who engages in an average amount of activity.

3. Read the results of scientific studies and assess the usefulness of the nutritional supplement for the activities you engage in.

Introduction to Sports Medicine Answer Key – Unit 2

Section 2.1

1. The cardiovascular system is comprised of the heart, the arteries, the veins, and the capillaries.

2. Arteries are elastic and capable stretching to accommodate the pulse of blood as it exits the heart, and contracting to permit blood to flow or obstructing its passage. The arteries are partially responsible for blood pressure via their contractile property. They are capable of redirecting blood flow where it is most needed. They have a thick muscular layer. They carry blood away from the heart.

   Veins carry blood toward the heart. Veins consist of the same three layers as arteries. However in veins, the tunica media is much thinner. Veins exert little effect on blood pressure for this reason.

3. Capillaries are where oxygen is released into the tissues and CO_2 is picked up for return to the lungs. Nutrients are exchanged for metabolic waste products at the capillaries.

Section 2.2

1. An EKG is a recording of the electrical activity of the heart as it beats. An abnormal EKG can tell the physician where the heart has a problem.

2. Systolic blood pressure is the maximum pressure exerted by the blood against the vasculature which occurs at the peak of ventricular contraction. Diastolic blood pressure is the minimum pressure exerted by the blood against the vasculature which occurs at the peak of ventricular relaxation.

3. The doctor applies pressure to a fingernail until the tissue blanches, then measures how long it takes for the color to return to the nail bed. A refill time of over two minutes may indicate PVD.

Section 2.3

1. The respiratory system consists of the lungs, the bronchi, the trachea, larynx, pharynx, and nasal passages.

2. The alveoli increase the surface area over which gasses can be exchanged and are the site of oxygen and carbon dioxide exchange.

3. Angiotensin I is converted into angiotensin II in the lungs. Angiotensin II causes the blood vessels to constrict, raising blood pressure.

Section 2.4

1. If the ratio is large, the lungs are capable of moving air easily. If the ratio is small, the lungs are having difficulty moving air, indicating an obstruction or constricted airways.

2. The MVV test provides the physician with information about the strength and function of the muscles responsible for breathing, the elasticity of the lungs, and airway resistance.

3. Males tend to have greater lung capacity than females, even when matched for height and weight. Increasing age tends to reduce elasticity, and thus capacity, of the lungs.

Section 2.5

1. The bones provide the body with shape and support, serve as a reservoir for Ca, and are home for the hematopoietic stem cells.

2. The ligaments serve to tie the bones together at the joints and stabilize the joint so that it only moves in the desired direction. Tendons connect the muscles to the bones and transmit muscular force.

3. The axial elements include the bones of the skull, vertebral column, ribs, and sternum. The appendicular elements include the bones of the arms, legs, hands, feet, the pelvic girdle, and the pectoral girdle.

Section 2.6

1. Cortical bone is composed of densely packed columns of osteons and serves as the hard outer layer of a bone. Cancellous bone fills the less dense interior of the bones with tiny strut-like bridges called trabeculae. Cancellous bone is home to the red bone marrow where hematopoietic stem cells reside, and the majority of the arteries and veins within the bone.

2. Cortical bone and cancellous bone provide structure and support to the body, provide levers upon which the muscles can act to move the body, protect the vital organs, and serve as a storage depot for minerals.

3. Osteoporosis is a reduction in bone density as a result of calcium loss in the bone. The stresses athletes place on their bones can cause them to fracture even in the absence of a blow if the bones are not dense and strong. In the case of athletes with low bone densities, even the impact of landing after a jump can result in a bone fracture. Many female athletes suffer from osteoporosis because of a combination of excessive exercise and inadequate nutrition.

Section 2.7

1. In sports medicine, the Stress-Strain curve is used to measure the ability of bones, ligaments, and tendons to bear the loads placed upon them by athletic competition. Trainers use their knowledge of the Stress-Strain curve to design appropriate training programs so that athletes' ligaments and tendons have a chance to adapt to the stresses being placed upon them gradually. Sports equipment manufacturers calculate the forces being generated against bones and other body structures to design protective gear that dissipates the force of the blow sufficiently to prevent broken bones.

2. The yield strength of a sample is the strain the sample can support without deforming plastically. The ultimate strength of a sample is the maximum stress it can bear when subjected to tension, compression, or shearing.

3. For brittle objects such as glass, any deformation results in rupture, but the object can be put back together as it was before rupture. Non-brittle objects undergo strain-hardening, necking, and ultimately rupture in such a way that they can never regain their original configuration.

Section 2.8

1. A typical joint is composed of bone, cartilage, ligaments, tendons, the joint capsule, the synovial membrane, and synovial fluid.

2. In a first-class lever, the fulcrum is located between the force and the load. A first class lever in the body would be the elbow joint of the arm extending because of the triceps muscle. In a second-class lever, the load is between the fulcrum and the applied force. A second class lever in the body would be the calf muscle, or gastrocnemius, flexing the foot.

3. In a first-class lever, the fulcrum is located between the force and the load. A first class lever in the body would be the elbow joint of the arm extending because of the triceps muscle. In a third-class lever, the force is applied between the fulcrum and the load. Flexing of the elbow by the biceps muscle is an example of a third class lever in the body.

Section 2.9

1. The muscular system is composed of the specialized contractile cells called myocytes which make movement of the body and within the body possible.

2. Smooth muscle is not under voluntary control. Smooth muscle cells are spindle-shaped. The nucleus of smooth muscle cells is usually located in the center of the cell. The actin and myosin chains are not arranged in any specific pattern within the cell. Smooth muscle has the ability to contract when something stretches the tissue.

   Striated muscle is under voluntary control by the central nervous system. Myofibers are multinucleate cells whose multiple nuclei are located just beneath the plasma membrane. Myofibers contain many mitochondria. Myofibers are packed densely with myofibrils, the proteins arranged as a long series of individual sarcomeres, the special functional unit of striated muscle.

3. Like striated muscle, cardiac muscle is striated in appearance. Similar to striated muscle, cardiomyocytes contain many mitochondria.

Section 2.10

1. The CNS is composed of the brain and the spinal cord. The brain and spinal cord are composed of neurons and glia, including oligodendrocytes and astrocytes.

2. The brain directly innervates the body via the twelve cranial nerves: the olfactory nerve, optic nerve, oculomotor nerve, trochlear nerve, abducens nerve, trigeminal nerve, facial nerve, vestibulochoclear nerve, glossopharyngeal nerve, vagus nerve, accessory nerve, and the hypoglossal nerve.

3. Reflexes are actions that occur almost instantly, that are often executed by voluntary muscles, and that are not under voluntary control. These actions are controlled within the spinal cord. A reflex arc occurs when an afferent sensory neuron stimulates an efferent motor neuron within the spinal cord to generate movement. The stimulus is relayed to the brain, but by the time the brain has registered the stimulus, the body has already moved.

Section 2.11

1. The FIT principle is a tool used by trainers to help individuals and athletes develop training programs to reach their goals. FIT stands for frequency, intensity, and time.

2. Exercise causes damage to the muscle cells, tendons, and ligaments of the body. The body repairs the damage and at the same time increases the size of the muscle or improves its aerobic capacity. The body strengthens ligaments, tendons, and bones. The body must have sufficient time to effect these repairs. High intensity or long duration exercise performed too frequently will result in weakening of the muscles, loss of muscle mass, and damage to the ligaments and tendons.

3. Exercise intensity is then calculated as a percentage of the maximum heart rate. High intensity aerobic workouts generally utilize a heart rate that is 80 to 90% of maximum, moderate intensity workouts use between 70 and 80%, and low intensity workouts use between 60 and 70% as their target heart rates.

Section 2.12

1. Power is measured in Watts (W) = Force (in Newtons) × distance (in meters) ÷ time (in seconds).

    2 N × 2 m / 10 sec = 0.4 W

2. Athletes use strength training with weights, plyometrics, and speed training elements in their workout regimens to increase power. Strength training increases overall strength which is half of power generation. Plyometrics and speed training increase the speed with which the strength can be applied.

3. Endurance training focuses on low to moderate intensity exercises performed for long periods of time to improve the efficiency of the muscle. Endurance training includes improvements in the efficiency of the cardiovascular system to carry oxygen and nutrients to the muscles and remove waste products. Strength training focuses on high intensity exercises performed over short time frames to increase the diameter of the muscles, the number of myofilaments in the muscle, and the density of the connective tissue surrounding the muscles. Strength training improves the anaerobic capabilities of the muscles.

Section 2.13

1. Aerobic conditioning is physical training which improves the body's ability to take in, distribute, and use oxygen during exercise.

2. Anaerobic conditioning stimulates improvement in the muscles' anaerobic metabolic system and the muscles' ability to recover from oxygen debt.

3. Interval training improves the body's ability to recover from anaerobic activity, improves anaerobic metabolism, and increases strength.

Section 2.14

1. A rep is a single exercise movement from start to finish. A set is a group of repetitions.

2. By varying the number of reps and sets, athletes can achieve very different goals using the same exercises.

3. To train for strength, an athlete will use heavy weights, low reps, and low to moderate numbers of sets. Endurance training typically utilizes lighter weights and higher reps and sets.

Section 2.15

1. Thibaudeau's six training methods are the Ballistic method, the Speed- strength method, the Strength-speed method, the Controlled repetition method, the Maximal method, and the Supra-maximal method. The ballistic method involves "throwing" the weight, hence the name ballistic. The Speed-strength method utilizes light weights, and typically involves sports- related movements. Acceleration and strength are equally important in the Strength-speed method. The Controlled repetition method is the classic bodybuilding method of heavy weights and isolation of specific muscle groups, coupled with controlled, relatively slow movements. The Maximal method combines maximum weight lifting, eccentric exercises, and isometric exercises to rapidly increase muscular strength. The Supra-maximal method must be used with extreme care. The athlete will be lifting loads in excess of his maximum capability.

2. Force production involves overcoming the inertia of an object, then accelerate its mass. How rapidly that mass is moved is a function of the ability to generate force. By increasing the speed with which an athlete can accelerate the mass, trainers can increase the athlete's strength without increasing the weight she must move, i.e., her force production.

3. Supra-maximal loads are lifted eccentrically, the athlete uses improper form to get past the sticking point, or the athlete does not use a complete range of motion for the exercise.

Introduction to Sports Medicine Answer Key – Unit 3

Section 3.1

1. A focal brain injury is an injury to the brain that is limited to a specific area of the brain. There is a focal point where the injury occurred and the damage was done.

2. There are four types of diffuse brain injury: diffuse vascular injury, diffuse swelling, diffuse hypoxic/anoxic/ ischemic injury, and diffuse axonal injury.

3. A concussion is a brain injury that results from a blow to the head, violent shaking of the head, gunshots, and whiplash injuries. Concussions are the mildest form of brain injury, but are nonetheless very serious. Concussions are difficult to diagnose.

Section 3.2

1. Spinal cord injuries can be complete, resulting in complete loss of sensation and control on both sides of the body below the injury, or incomplete, permitting some level of sensation and control below the injury.

2. Spinal cord injuries can occur at the Cervical, Thoracic, Lumbar, and Sacral levels.

3. Axial loading refers to placing a load on the second vertebra of the spinal column, the axis, usually as a result of a blow to the top of the head. These injuries are most common in young athletes, especially in football, diving, rugby, and gymnastics. Axial loading occurs when the spine is straightened by lowering the head slightly. This position prevents the ligaments, tendons, and muscles from absorbing the impact and transmits the force to the vertebra. The vertebra can be crushed, or it can slide forward, backward or laterally to shear the spinal cord.

Section 3.3

1. Emergency responders to spinal cord injury must remember the ABC's of emergency medicine: Airway, Breathing, Circulation. The spine should be completely immobilized; the neck should be secured with a cervical hard collar and the patient should be securely immobilized on a hard backboard for transportation to the hospital.

2. The doctor should collect a complete history of the injury and complete a neurological assessment, followed by X-rays, CT scans, or MRI of the spine.

3. The doctor should provide analgesic medications and high doses of methylprednisolone within 8 hours of injury. Belts, keys, wallets, and other hard objects should be removed from the patient, and portions of the body that will be in contact with surfaces should be padded. Patients should be turned ever 1-2 hours to limit the likelihood of pressure necrosis. Spinal cord injury patients must be watched carefully for lung problems and poor or no breathing, hypothermia, pneumonia, and urinary tract infections.

Section 3.4

1. The bones composing the shoulder are the scapula, humerus, and clavicle.

2. The muscles and tendons of the rotator cuff are the supraspinatus, subscapularis, infraspinatus, and teres minor.

3. An orthopedic physician will perform a reduction. The shoulder should be treated with rest, ice, and non-steroidal anti-inflammatory medication.

Section 3.5

1. The bones that compose the elbow joint are the radius, ulna, and humerus.

2. The ligaments of the elbow are the ulnar collateral ligament, radial collateral ligament, and the annular ligament.

3. Rest, ice, compression, elevation, and physical therapy can alleviate tennis elbow.

Section 3.6

1. The eight carpal bones are the scaphoid, lunate, triquetrum, trapezium, trapezoid, capitate, hamate, and pisiform bones.

2. The ligaments of the wrist are the ulnar collateral ligament, radial collateral ligament, and transverse carpal ligament. The wrist serves as a passageway for the flexor tendons and the extensor tendons.

3. A sprain is an injury to the ligament in which it is stretched beyond its ability to return to its original shape. Sprains are treated using RICE, rest, ice, elevation, and compression. Anti-inflammatory medications such as aspirin, acetaminophen, ibuprofen, or naproxen can help reduce the swelling and pain caused by a sprain.

Section 3.7

1. The hand is made up of the metacarpal bones and the phalanges.

2. The phalanges are stabilized by collateral ligaments and the volar plate. The muscles of the hand include the thenar muscle, the hypothenal muscles, the interosseous muscles, and the lumbrical muscles.

3. In a study of hospital emergency rooms, lacerations, bruises, fractures, and infections, are the most common injuries of the hand in that order.

Section 3.8

1. The curves help to distribute the forces acting on the spine across the entire spinal column rather than at the site at which the force is applied. Proper curvature of the spine is important for correct movement of the extremities, proper breathing, and proper digestion.

2. Lordosis is an exaggerated inward curvature of the lumbar spine. Lordosis causes lower back pain, pushes the hips backward, and makes walking and running difficult. Kyphosis is a curvature of the cervical and thoracic vertebrae that rounds the back and lowers the head. Kyphosis causes pain, makes breathing difficult, compresses the viscera, and slows the passage of food through the digestive tract. Scoliosis is a lateral curvature of the vertebral column. Patients may suffer from pain, uneven hips, shoulders, and/or ribs, or slower neural responses.

3. A slipped disc does not really slip. Instead, the disc tears, and the gel-like material inside leaks out and pushes against the spinal cord. Slipped discs are usually caused by improperly lifting heavy or bulky items, especially when turning or twisting.

Section 3.9

1. The hip is a sturdy ball and socket joint between the femur and the pelvis. The hip provides support and balance to the body while standing and during locomotion. The hip joint is much more stable than the shoulder, but incapable of as wide a range of motion as the shoulder. The hip joint is surrounded by a joint capsule, which is composed of an outer fibrous connective tissue layer and the inner synovial membrane. Articular cartilage covers the end of the femur and the inner surface of the hip socket. There are five ligaments at the hip joint; four extracapsular ligaments and one intracapsular ligament. The extracapsular ligaments of the hip are the iliofemoral, ischiofemoral, pubofemoral, and zona orbicularis ligaments. The iliofemoral ligament is the strongest ligament in the body, and it stabilizes the body when it is in an upright position. The ischiofemoral ligament prevents rotation of the leg toward the center of the body. The pubofemoral ligament prevents the legs from "splitting". The zona orbicularis forms a collar around the femoral head to prevent it slipping backward out of the joint, similar to a buttonhole. The ligamentum teres is the intracapsular ligament. It connects the head of the femur to the interior of the hip socket to prevent hip dislocation.

2. Alterations of the movement of the hips in response to injury alter all of the movements in the body. The repositioning of the hip to avoid pain or to move an injured leg places stress on the muscles of the lower back and causes misalignment of the vertebrae, changes posture, the angle of the shoulders, affecting the movement of the arms. The femur may rotate inward or outward, changing the angle with which the femur meets the tibia and fibula in the knee and placing additional stresses on the knee. The change in the angle of the knee changes the angle with which the tibia and fibula meet the tarsal bones of the ankle. Additional new stresses are placed on the ankle.

3. Hip stress fracture is treated with rest and ice, but pain medications should be avoided. This is to make sure painful activities which continue to damage the bone are avoided. Hip osteonecrosis usually requires total hip replacement. Labral tear is treated with rest, anti-inflammatory medications, and physical therapy. Surgery can be used in severe or unresponsive cases. Dislocation is treated by manipulating the femoral head back into the socket after anaesthetizing the patient. Physical therapy for two to three months is usually required.

Section 3.10

1. The knee is comprised of four bones, the femur, or thigh bone, tibia, or shin bone, fibula, which runs alongside the tibia, and the patella, or knee cap.

2. The two medial collateral ligaments, the anterior cruciate ligament and posterior cruciate ligament, stabilize the joint. The collateral ligaments protect against lateral movement of the knee. The anterior cruciate ligament prevents the femur from sliding forward on the tibia. The posterior cruciate ligament prevents the femur from sliding backward on the tibia.

3. The patella is held in place by the tendons of the four heads of the quadriceps muscle and the patellar tendon. The quadriceps and the hamstrings help hold the knee in place. The quadriceps extend the knee. The hamstrings are responsible for flexing the knee.

Section 3.11

1. Knee cartilage wears away due to overuse, injuries, or excessive weight gain resulting in osteoarthritis. The bones begin to rub against one another directly. Over-the-counter anti-inflammatory medications and pain relievers can be used to reduce the pain and swelling. Weight loss can reduce the severity of osteoarthritis. Exercises that improve the strength of the muscles around the knee can improve joint stability and reduce friction. Knee replacement surgery is becoming common in severe cases of osteoarthritis.

2. Ligament injuries are sprains or more severe tears. Anterior cruciate ligament (ACL) sprains and tears are usually caused by a twisting motion. Posterior cruciate ligament sprains (PCL) and tears are caused by a blow to the leg that forces the knee forward. Sprains and tears of the collateral ligaments are usually caused by a blow to the outside of the knee. Ligament injuries are treated with ice to reduce the swelling. A brace and exercise therapies to strengthen the muscles help stabilize the knee and reduce the strain on the ligaments. In severe cases, surgery is required to repair the ligaments.

3. Tendons are typically injured by overuse. Tendonitis causes pain and swelling. The result is a weakened tendon. Tendons that are overused and weakened are susceptible to stretching or tearing. In older people, tendons can be torn while trying to land during a fall. Tendonitis is treated with rest, ice, compression, and elevation. Over- the-counter anti-inflammatory medications help reduce the swelling. In the case of a ruptured tendon, surgery will be required.

Section 3.12

1. The ankle is really made up of two joints, the subtalar joint, and the true ankle joint. The true ankle joint includes the tibia and fibula of the lower leg with the talus. The true ankle joint permits flexion and extension of the foot. The subtalar joint includes the talus and the calcaneus.

2. The anterior and posterior tibiofibular ligaments bind the tibia and fibula to one another. The anterior and posterior talofibular ligaments, and calcenofibular ligament, provide lateral stability to the ankle. The deltoid ligament binds the inside surface of the fibula to the inside surface of the talus to prevent the ankle from rolling inward.

3. A broken ankle is an injury to the bones of the ankle. While a broken ankle is extremely painful, it is not uncommon for the patient to be capable of walking on it. A sprain is a ligament injury. Sprains are so painful the patient will not be able to walk on the injured foot.

Section 3.13

1. The bones of the feet include five tarsal bones, navicular bone, the cuboidal bone, and the first, second, and third cuneiform bones, five metatarsal bones, and five phalanges.

2. Heel spurs are an overuse injury in which a bony outgrowth occurs where a chronically inflamed tendon or ligament attaches to the bone. Heel spurs can be quite painful. Treatment for heel spurs includes taping the injured area to reduce use, anti- inflammatory medication, and physical therapy. When these fail, the heel spur is removed surgically.

3. Some of the tendons attach muscles found within the foot to the bones of the foot. These muscles and tendons are called intrinsic muscles and intrinsic tendons, because they are intrinsic to, or part of, the foot. Tendons also reach the foot from muscles of the lower leg, especially the calf muscles. These tendons and muscles are referred to as extrinsic muscles and tendons, because they arise outside the foot itself.

Section 3.14

1. Osteoarthritis is a condition in which the articular cartilage of the joint on the end of the bone has been worn away by disease, overuse, or injury. The result is that the bones grind on one another rather than gliding smoothly past one another when the joint is used. Movement is painful, and often the range of motion of the joint becomes limited.

2. Treatment for osteoarthritis typically begins with NSAIDS to reduce the immune response, reduce the inflammation, and alleviate the pain of osteoarthritis in most cases. When NSAIDS are not enough, doctors may resort to using corticosteroids, but the benefits of steroids for osteoarthritis treatment are controversial. Joint replacement surgery is the last resort for treatment of osteoarthritis. Hips, knees, and shoulders can be replaced with artificial joints.

3. Running causes overuse injuries to the ankles, knees, hips, and lower spine. The constant jarring impact of the foot hitting the ground compresses the joints, weakens the ligaments, and damages the cartilage. Weakened ligaments destabilize the joint and permit contact between the ends of the bones. Over time, the articular cartilage of the joint is worn down. The result is osteoarthritis. Football injuries tend to cause osteoarthritis via trauma, directly damaging the cartilage. Other injuries cause ligament damage, destabilizing the joint, and allowing the articular cartilage of the bones to rub against one another. Over time, the articular cartilage can wear away, resulting in osteoarthritis.

Section 3.15

1. The core muscles of the abdomen include the rectus abdominus, external obliques, internal obliques, and transverse abdominus. The core muscles of the lower back include the longissimus thoracis, quadrates lumborum, multifidus, and ilio-costalis lumborum.

2. The core stabilizes the body during movement by aligning the hips, spine, and ribs so that the body maintains its balance. It also initiates movements of the extremities by moving the hip to begin leg movements, or transferring power from the hips and legs to the arms for throwing, swinging, or striking motions.

4. The abdominal muscles must keep the viscera in place and dissipate the force of any impacts to the abdomen. The rectus abdominus, commonly called the "six-pack" muscles, tighten to absorb and dissipate the force of a blow.

www.ingramcontent.com/pod-product-compliance
Lightning Source LLC
Chambersburg PA
CBHW080241180526
45167CB00006B/2370